RHEUMATOID ARTHRITIS COOKBOOK FOR NEWLY DIAGNOSED

Anti-Inflammatory Diet Recipes for Fighting Flares and Relief of Joint Pain

Mary J. Barnes RDN

ACKNOWLEDGMENT

This cookbook wouldn't exist without so many people's amazing support and encouragement.

First of all, I want to say a huge thank you to my husband, Joan, and my kids, Clara and Jimmy. Your love, patience, and understanding have been my rock throughout this whole process. Thank you for cheering me on, trying all those recipes, and helping me find the humorous side of things, even when things were hard.

To everyone else fighting RA: Your strength and resilience inspire me daily. Thank you for sharing your stories, challenging times, and victories. This book is for you.

I'm so grateful to my rheumatologist, Dr. Elizabeth Ander, for her kind care and constant support. Your knowledge and guidance have been incredibly helpful in managing my RA and getting my life back.

To my dear friend and colleague, Olivia Miller, RDN, thank you for your amazing insights and feedback on the recipes in this book. Your passion for nutrition and helping others is truly inspiring.

I also want to say a big thank you to the team at Mary J. Barnes, RDN, especially Joan K. Barnes PhD, for believing in this project and making it happen. Your professionalism, excitement, and creative vision have been vital in making this cookbook a reality.

Lastly, I'm thankful for all the researchers, healthcare professionals, and advocates who are working so hard to improve the lives of people with RA. Your dedication gives us all hope for a better future.

Thank you, from the bottom of my heart.

WHY THIS BOOK?

The day my doctor said I had "rheumatoid arthritis," my world felt like it turned upside down. It was like a sudden storm of feelings – confusion, fear, and a deep sadness for what I thought I had lost. I wasn't ready for any of this. I felt lost, trying to find something to hold onto in a sea of confusing medical words and advice that didn't make sense together.

Even though I'm a registered dietitian nutritionist and know food can heal and make us strong, I had trouble finding good information about how to eat to manage my new life with RA. The cookbooks I found were full of ingredients I didn't know and recipes that seemed way too hard, and they didn't seem to understand the special problems people with RA face.

That's when I started thinking about making this cookbook.

I wanted to make something that I needed when I was first diagnosed – a guide that spoke to my heart and my head, a friend on this journey, not just a list of recipes.

"Rheumatoid Arthritis Cookbook for Newly Diagnosed" comes from my own life and my passion for helping others through food. It's made with love and filled with recipes that are not only tasty and help fight inflammation but also easy to make, even on days when your joints hurt. It's a book that understands how emotional it is to be newly diagnosed, and it offers comfort, hope, and practical things you can do.

Whether you're a great cook or just starting, cooking for yourself or your family, you'll find recipes here that work for you and what you like to eat. More importantly, you'll find a group of people who understand and a reminder that you're not alone on this journey.

I hope this cookbook becomes a close friend in your kitchen, inspiring and nourishing you as you face the challenges of living with RA. I hope it gives you the power to take control of your health, find your joy again, and enjoy the simple happiness of a tasty, healing meal.

With warmth and understanding,

TABLE OF CONTENTS

HOW TO USE THIS COOKBOOK

1. **Start at the Beginning:** If RA or anti-inflammatory eating is new to you, start with the first few chapters. They'll teach you the basics about RA and how food can help you feel better.

2. **Check Out the Recipes:** Look through the different chapters to find recipes you'll enjoy and that fit your dietary needs. Each recipe has clear instructions, nutrition facts, and ideas for changing things up.

3. **Think About Your Needs:** Pay attention to the recipe notes and symbols that show if a recipe is gluten-free, vegan, or can be made ahead of time. Pick recipes that work for your diet and how much energy you have.

4. **Plan Ahead:** Use the meal planning and prep tips in the Chapter so you have healthy meals ready even on busy days.

5. **Listen to Your Body:** Everyone with RA is different. If you notice certain foods make your symptoms worse, feel free to change the recipes or try something else.

6. **Have Fun in the Kitchen:** Cooking should be enjoyable! Be creative and adjust the recipes to your liking.

7. **Enjoy the Journey:** Managing RA is an ongoing process. This cookbook is here to help you every step of the way, with yummy and easy recipes to nourish your body and mind.

More Helpful Tips:

a) **Eat Mostly Whole Foods:** Choose fresh, unprocessed ingredients as much as possible.

b) **Drink Plenty of Water:** Stay hydrated throughout the day to help your joints and overall health.

c) **Manage Stress:** Do things that help you relax, like gentle exercise, meditation, or spending time in nature.

d) **Celebrate Your Success:** Every step you take to manage your RA is a win. Celebrate your progress and be kind to yourself.

INTRODUCTION

Being told you have rheumatoid arthritis (RA) is a tough moment—it's like a sudden wake-up call that your body, which you used to rely on for everything, is now fighting a battle you didn't expect.

The first shock, the waves of fear and not knowing what will happen, the scary thought of your life being changed forever—these feelings are very familiar to people who've been told, "You have rheumatoid arthritis." It can feel like a heavy blanket, obscuring the future and leaving you feeling lost and alone.

But even in the darkness, there's a little bit of hope. More and more research is showing that what we choose to eat can make a big difference in how this long-term illness affects us. The food we eat can either make the inflammation worse or act like a gentle healer, making the pain less and helping us get better.

That's where *"The Rheumatoid Arthritis Cookbook for the Newly Diagnosed"* comes in, shining a light on you who are just starting to deal with RA. It's more than just recipes—but is a helping hand, proof that food can change things. Inside this cookbook, you'll find lots of information about RA, explained clearly and simply. We'll make the science behind inflammation easy to understand, see how food and the disease are connected, and give you the tools to make smart choices about what you eat.

But this isn't about giving up things you love or feeling restricted. Instead, it's about celebrating the tasty flavors and healthy ingredients that can help you feel better and stronger. We'll introduce you to lots of foods that fight inflammation, from colorful fruits and vegetables to good fats and lean proteins. You'll learn how to use these ingredients in your everyday meals, making dishes that are both yummy and good for you.

Our recipes are made with you in mind. We know that living with RA can make things difficult in the kitchen, such as joint pain, tiredness, or difficulty moving around. That's why we focused on making things straightforward to prepare, so you can make healthy and satisfying meals without too much effort. But more than just the practical stuff, this cookbook is also meant to inspire and encourage you. We'll share stories of people who have successfully managed their RA by changing their diet, showing you what's possible. You'll learn how food can be a powerful helper in your journey to feeling better and being healthy.

Benefits Of Rheumatoid Arthritis Cookbook for Newly Diagnosed:

1. **Discover the Healing Power of Food:** Learn how certain foods can fight inflammation and make your RA symptoms less severe.

2. **Enjoy Delicious and Easy Recipes:** Make tasty meals that are simple to prepare, even on days when your joints hurt.

3. **Specifically for Newly Diagnosed Individuals:** Find clear explanations and helpful tips for dealing with the early stages of RA.

4. **Empowerment and Support:** Feel more confident in managing your condition by making informed choices about what you eat.

5. **Improved Quality of Life:** Experience less pain, more energy, easy exercises, and a greater sense of control over your health.

Jessica is a lively young woman in her early thirties who lived a full and energetic life. She balanced a busy job with being a mom, always on the move, and seemingly unstoppable. But then, things started to change a little. She felt a constant ache in her hands, a stiffness in her joints that didn't go away even after a wonderful night's sleep.

At first, she thought these were just normal things that happen when you're busy. But as the weeks turned into months, the pain got worse, spreading to her wrists, knees, and ankles. Simple things she used to do without thinking, like tying her shoes or opening a jar, became really hard. She was always tired, drained, and felt like she couldn't do anything.

After seeing a few doctors and getting some tests, she was diagnosed with rheumatoid arthritis. Jessica's world fell apart. The future she had imagined, full of travel, adventure, and endless possibilities, now seemed uncertain and out of reach.

The medicine she was given helped a little, but the side effects were bad, making her feel even worse. She wanted to feel like she had some control—a way to actively help herself get better.

That's when she found out about an anti-inflammatory diet. The idea of managing her RA with food interested her, so she started doing research, reading books and articles, and trying new things in the kitchen.

It was challenging at first to change her habits. Old ways are difficult to break, and she wanted to eat comfort foods. But with each small change, Jessica felt stronger and more in control. She discovered new tastes, learned to appreciate simple, whole foods, and found joy in making healthy meals for herself and her family.

As she kept up with the anti-inflammatory way of eating, Jessica noticed a slow but big change in how she felt. The joint pain that used to bother her all the time started to get better. She wasn't as tired anymore and had more energy. She was able to go back to doing a lot of the things she loved, from playing with her son to working on her career goals.

Jessica's story shows us that we're not helpless when faced with difficult situations. Even with a chronic illness like RA, we can make choices that help us be healthy. Food can be a powerful way to heal and a source of comfort and strength.

This cookbook is an invitation for you to start your journey of change. Let it be your guide as you deal with the challenges of RA, helping you make smart choices, enjoy delicious food, and feel alive again.

Note the hope is here, with knowledge, hard work, and a little bit of creativity in the kitchen, you can create a life that is rich, fulfilling, and free from the limitations of RA

CHAPTER 1:
UNDERSTANDING RHEUMATOID ARTHRITIS & ROLE OF NUTRITION

Some wise words were spoken a long time ago, and still hold today when we think about rheumatoid arthritis (RA) and how important food is for managing it. RA is a disease where the body's immune system attacks itself, causing long-term inflammation in the joints. It affects millions of people around the world and can be very painful and make it hard to do things. While doctors and medicine are important for treating RA, we shouldn't forget about the power of food.

"Let food be thy medicine and medicine be thy food." - **Hippocrates**

RA isn't just about the joints; it's a problem with inflammation that can affect different parts of the body. The immune system, which is supposed to protect us from bad things, mistakenly attacks the lining of the joints, causing pain, swelling, stiffness, and even damage to the joints. Over time, RA can make it challenging to live your life the way you want, limiting how you move, making everyday tasks difficult, and even leading to feeling sad or anxious.

Who's More Likely to Get Rheumatoid Arthritis?

1. **Gender:** Women are more likely to develop it than men.

2. **Age:** It can happen at any age but is most common in middle age.

3. **Family History:** Your risk increases if a family member has RA.

4. **Smoking:** Smoking significantly raises your risk, especially if you're genetically predisposed. It can also worsen the disease.

5. **Obesity:** Being overweight slightly increases your risk.

Common Symptoms

1. Joint pain, tenderness, swelling, or stiffness lasting at least six weeks.

2. Morning stiffness lasting 30 minutes or more.

3. Multiple joints are affected, often starting with smaller joints like wrists, fingers, and toes.

4. The same joints on both sides of the body are usually involved.

How RA Affects Your Health

1. **Eyes:** Dryness, discomfort, inflammation, redness, sensitivity to light, and blurred vision.

2. **Mouth:** Dryness, gum inflammation, irritation, and infections.

3. **Skin:** Small bumps under the skin over bony areas (rheumatoid nodules).

4. **Lungs:** Inflammation and scarring can lead to shortness of breath and lung disease.

5. **Blood Vessels:** Inflammation can damage nerves, skin, and organs.

6. **Blood:** Reduced red blood cell count (anemia).

7. **Heart:** Inflammation can affect the heart muscle and surrounding tissues.

8. **Weight:** Joint pain can make exercise difficult, leading to weight gain, which increases the risk of other health problems like high cholesterol, diabetes, heart disease, and high blood pressure.

We don't know exactly what causes RA, but it's probably a mix of things in our genes and things in our environment. One of the most important things we can change is our diet, even though we can't change our genes.

New research is showing that what we eat can have a big effect on the inflammation that causes RA. Some foods can trigger or make inflammation worse, while others have special properties that can calm down the immune system and make symptoms better. By making healthy choices about what to eat, people with RA can take an active role in their healing and feel more in control of their condition.

The anti-inflammatory diet is a crucial component of nutrition for RA. It focuses on whole, unprocessed foods that are full of antioxidants, vitamins, minerals, and omega-3 fatty acids. These nutrients work together to fight inflammation, protect the joints, and make you feel healthier overall.

Fruits and vegetables are the most important anti-inflammatory foods because of their bright colors and flavors. They contain many antioxidants, which stop harmful things from happening in the body and protect cells from damage. Berries are especially effective at fighting inflammation because they have high levels of anthocyanins, powerful antioxidants that give berries their bright colors. Leafy greens, like spinach and kale, are also full of nutrients that help the immune system and reduce inflammation.

Fatty fish, like salmon, tuna, and sardines, are also essential for people with RA. They have lots of omega-3 fatty acids, which have been shown to reduce inflammation, make joints move better, and even mean you might need less medicine. You can also get omega-3s from plants, like flaxseeds, chia seeds, and walnuts.

Whole grains, like brown rice, quinoa, and oats, give you steady energy and fiber, which is good for your gut and helps control inflammation. Refined grains, on the other hand, should be limited because they can cause spikes in blood sugar and make inflammation worse.

Nuts and seeds are a good source of healthy fats, protein, and fiber. Almonds, walnuts, and pumpkin seeds are especially good for RA because they fight inflammation.

Legumes, like lentils, beans, and chickpeas, are packed with plant-based protein and fiber. They also have lots of antioxidants and other nutrients that help the immune system and reduce inflammation.

Herbs and spices, which are often forgotten about, are strong helpers in the fight against inflammation. Turmeric, ginger, garlic, and cinnamon are just a few examples of spices that have powerful anti-inflammatory properties. Adding these to your food can make it taste better and help you heal.

While the anti-inflammatory diet focuses mostly on plant-based foods, that doesn't mean you can't eat any animal products. Lean protein, like chicken, turkey, and fish, can be eaten in moderation. But it's important to choose good-quality options and limit red meat and processed meats, which can make inflammation worse.

It's also important to pay attention to what you're not eating. Highly processed foods, full of added sugars, harmful fats, and artificial ingredients, can trigger inflammation and make RA symptoms worse. Sugary drinks, refined grains, and fried foods should be limited or avoided completely. The power of food to heal and change things is real. People with RA can see a big improvement in how they feel when they eat an anti-inflammatory diet. Less pain, better movement, more energy, and feeling more in control are just some of the possible benefits.

However, the impact of changing your diet goes beyond the physical. As you nourish your body with healthy, anti-inflammatory foods, you'll also feel better mentally and emotionally. Cooking and sharing meals can bring you joy and connect you with others, creating a sense of community and belonging. You'll rediscover the pleasure of enjoying each bite, mindful of the nourishment it provides and the positive effect it has on your health.

This isn't a quick fix or a magic solution. Managing RA takes a lot of different things, including medicine, lifestyle changes, and support from family and friends. But by using the power of food, you can take an active role in your healing and create a life that is full of joy, satisfaction, and free from the limitations of RA.

Managing Rheumatoid Arthritis

1. **Healthy Eating:** A balanced diet with the right amount of each food group helps you feel good and maintain a healthy weight.

2. **Stay Active:** implementing movement exercises into your daily routine, even if it's just taking the stairs or parking further away.

3. **Balance Activity and Rest:** While staying active is important, rest is crucial during flares. It reduces inflammation and fatigue.

4. **Hot and Cold Treatments:** Use heat for stiff joints and tired muscles, and cold for acute pain and swelling.

5. **Topical Products:** Creams, gels, and patches can provide temporary relief for joint and muscle pain.

6. **Stress Reduction and Complementary Therapies:** Try meditation, deep breathing, massage, or acupuncture to manage stress and pain.

7. **Supplements:** Curcumin/turmeric and omega-3 fish oil may help with RA symptoms, but talk to your doctor first.

Some Tips to Help You Make Dietary Adjustments For RA

1. **Start Small, Think Big:** Don't try to change everything at once. Begin by adding one or two new anti-inflammatory foods to your meals each day.

2. **Add Good, Don't Just Take Away Bad:** Instead of focusing on cutting out unhealthy foods, focus on adding more healthy ones. When your plate is full of nutritious choices, there's less room for the less healthy ones.

3. **One Swap at a Time:** Each week, replace one processed food with a whole-food alternative. For example, switch white rice for brown rice or sugary cereal for oatmeal with fruit and nuts.

4. **Plan and Prepare:** Make it easier on yourself by planning your meals and snacks ahead of time. This will help you avoid making unhealthy choices on the spot and make sure you have healthy options ready to go.

5. **Read Labels:** Be a smart shopper by reading food labels carefully. Look for products with few ingredients and avoid those with added sugars, unhealthy fats, and artificial stuff.

6. **Cook More Often:** Cooking your meals lets you control what goes into them and gives you a chance to try new flavors and textures.

7. **Find Healthy Substitutes:** Don't feel like you're missing out! There are lots of tasty and healthy alternatives to your favorite foods. Try new recipes and discover how fun it can be to cook with anti-inflammatory ingredients.

8. **Be Patient and Kind to Yourself:** Change takes time, and you might have some setbacks. Don't be too harsh on yourself if you slip up.

Date: _____

Monday:_____
_____
_____

Tuesday:_____
_____
_____

Wednesday:_____
_____
_____

Thursday:_____
_____
_____

Friday:_____
_____
_____

Saturday:_____
_____
_____

Sunday:_____
_____
_____

Exercise/Observation:_____
_____
_____
_____

CHAPTER 2:
GROCERY SHOPPING LIST FOR AN RA-FRIENDLY DIET

Produce:

1. **Dark Leafy Greens:**

- Arugula
- Collard greens
- Kale
- Lettuce (various types like romaine, butter lettuce)
- Spinach
- Swiss chard

2. **Root Vegetables:**

- Beets
- Carrots
- Celery root (celeriac)
- Parsnips
- Sweet potatoes

3. **Winter Squashes:**

- Acorn squash
- Butternut squash

4. **Other Vegetables:**

- Asparagus
- Broccoli
- Brussels sprouts
- Cabbage
- Cauliflower
- Eggplant
- Garlic
- Ginger
- Green beans
- Mushrooms (various types)
- Onions (red, yellow, white)
- Peppers (bell peppers, chili peppers)
- Radishes
- Zucchini

5. **Fruits:**

- Apples
- Bananas
- Blackberries
- Blueberries
- Cherries
- Clementines
- Grapefruit
- Guava
- Kiwi
- Lemons
- Limes

- Mangoes
- Melons (watermelon, cantaloupe, honeydew)
- Nectarines
- Oranges
- Papaya
- Peaches
- Pears
- Pineapple
- Plums
- Pomegranate arils
- Raspberries
- Strawberries
- Tangerines

Pantry Staples:

1. **Beans and Legumes:**

- Black beans
- Chickpeas
- Lentils

2. **Grains:**

- Brown rice
- Oats (steel-cut, rolled, or Irish)
- Quinoa
- Wild rice

3. **Nuts and Seeds:**

- Almonds
- Chia seeds
- Flaxseeds
- Pumpkin seeds
- Sesame seeds
- Sunflower seeds
- Walnuts

4. **Oils and Fats:**

- Avocado oil
- Extra virgin olive oil
- Flaxseed oil (store in the refrigerator)
- Ghee or butter (if tolerated)
- Nut butter (almond, cashew, etc.)
- Virgin coconut oil

5. **Spices and Herbs:**

- Basil
- Cayenne pepper
- Chili powder
- Cinnamon
- Cilantro
- Cloves
- Cumin
- Curry powder
- Dill
- Fennel
- Ginger
- Nutmeg
- Oregano

- Paprika
- Parsley
- Red pepper flakes
- Rosemary

- Sage
- Thyme
- Turmeric

Protein:

1. **Fish:**

- Halibut
- Salmon
- Trout

2. **Meat:**

- Beef (grass-fed, if possible)
- Chicken (boneless, skinless breasts or thighs)
- Ground turkey
- Lamb
- Pork (loin chops, tenderloin)
- Sausage (Italian, ensure low-fat and nitrate-free)

3. **Other Protein Sources:**

- Eggs
- Hummus
- Tofu

Dairy (if tolerated):

1. **Cheese:**

- Feta
- Goat cheese

2. **Yogurt:**

- Low-fat Greek yogurt

Additional:

1. Sweeteners (natural):

- Coconut sugar
- Maple syrup
- Molasses
- Stevia

2. **Other:**

- Almond flour
- Baking powder
- Baking soda
- Broth (chicken or vegetable)
- Chia seeds
- Coconut flakes
- Coconut milk
- Corn tortillas
- Dried fruit (unsweetened)
- Gluten-free flour blend
- Maple extract
- Nut milk (almond, cashew, etc.)
- Nutritional yeast
- Tahini
- Vanilla extract

- Vinegar (balsamic, apple cider, etc.)

Foods to Limit or Avoid on an RA Diet

Highly Processed Foods:

1. **Refined grains**: White bread, white pasta, pastries, cookies, cakes, crackers

2. **Sugary drinks**: Soda, sweetened juices, energy drinks

3. **Packaged snacks**: Chips, candy, cookies, processed meats (hot dogs, bacon)

4. **Fast food:** Burgers, fries, fried chicken

5. **Frozen meals:** Many contain high levels of sodium, unhealthy fats, and added sugars

6. **Breakfast cereals**: Many are highly processed and contain added sugars

Foods High in Saturated and Trans Fats:

1. **Red meat:** Limit consumption, especially fatty cuts

2. **Full-fat dairy products**: Choose low-fat or non-fat options

3. **Fried foods**: Limit deep-fried foods and those cooked in excessive oil

4. **Butter and margarine**: option for healthier fats like olive oil or avocado oil

Other Inflammatory Foods:

1. **Added sugars:** Limit sweets, desserts, and foods with added sugars

2. **Alcohol:** Consume in moderation, if at all

3. **Nightshade vegetables:** Some individuals with RA may find these trigger symptoms (tomatoes, potatoes, eggplants, peppers)

4. **Gluten:** If you have a gluten sensitivity or celiac disease, avoid gluten-containing foods

CHAPTER 3:
BREAKFAST DIET FOR RA

1. Fruit-and-Seed Breakfast Bars

These Fruit-and-Seed Breakfast Bars offer a delicious and nutritious way to start your day. Rich in anti-inflammatory ingredients like nuts, seeds, and fruits, they provide sustained energy and essential nutrients while being gentle on joints.

INGREDIENTS:

- 1 cup rolled oats (gluten-free if needed)
- 1/2 cup mixed nuts (almonds, walnuts, pecans)
- 1/2 cup mixed seeds (chia, flax, sunflower, pumpkin)
- 1/2 cup dried fruit (dates, cranberries, apricots)
- 1/4 cup honey or maple syrup
- 1/4 cup nut butter (almond, cashew, or sunflower seed)
- 1/4 cup coconut oil, melted
- 1 teaspoon vanilla extract
- Pinch of salt

PREPARATION METHODS:

1. Heat the oven to 350°F (175°C) and line an 8x8 inch baking pan with parchment paper.

2. In a large bowl, combine the oats, nuts, seeds, and dried fruit.

3. In a separate bowl, mix the honey or maple syrup, nut butter, coconut oil, vanilla extract, and salt.

4. Pour the wet ingredients over the dry ingredients and mix until well combined.

5. Press the mixture evenly into the prepared baking pan.

6. Bake for 20-25 minutes, or until golden brown.

7. Let cool completely in the pan before cutting into bars.

PREP TIPS:

1. To make the bars chewier, soak the dried fruit in hot water for 10 minutes before using.

2. For nut-free options, substitute the nuts with additional seeds or oats.

3. You can select the bars by adding different spices, such as cinnamon or cardamom.

4. Store the bars in an airtight container at room temperature for up to a week or in the refrigerator for up to two weeks.

NUTRITIONAL VALUES PER SERVING (1 BAR):

Calories: Approximately 200-250 calories (depending on ingredients) | Protein: 5-7 grams | Fiber: 4-6 grams | Fats: 10-15 grams

Serving Portion: 1 bar

Prep Time: 15 minutes

Cooking Time: 20-25 minutes

DIET RECIPE NOTE:

- This recipe is suitable for an RA diet as it is rich in anti-inflammatory ingredients and contains no refined sugars or unhealthy fats.

- It is naturally gluten-free if gluten-free oats are used.

- The recipe can be easily adapted to be vegan by using maple syrup instead of honey and vegan nut butter.

- If nightshades are a concern, ensure the dried fruit blend doesn't include goji berries.

2. Chia-Coconut Porridge

Chia-Coconut Porridge is a creamy and satisfying breakfast option that's rich in nutrients and anti-inflammatory benefits. The combination of chia seeds and coconut milk provides a healthy dose of omega-3 fatty acids, fiber, and antioxidants. This recipe is quick and easy to prepare, making it a great choice for busy mornings.

INGREDIENTS:

- 1/2 cup unsweetened coconut milk

- 1/4 cup water

- 3 tablespoons chia seeds

- 1 tablespoon shredded coconut (unsweetened)

- 1/2 teaspoon vanilla extract

- Optional toppings: fresh berries, sliced bananas, chopped nuts, a drizzle of honey or maple syrup (use sparingly)

PREPARATION METHOD:

1. In a bowl or jar, combine the coconut milk, water, chia seeds, shredded coconut, and vanilla extract.

2. Stir well to ensure all the chia seeds are evenly distributed.

3. Cover the bowl or jar and refrigerate overnight, or for at least 4 hours, until the mixture thickens into a porridge-like thickness.

4. In the morning, give the porridge a good stir.

5. Top with your desired toppings and enjoy!

PREP TIPS:

1. For a creamier texture, use full-fat coconut milk.

2. If you like a sweeter porridge, add a small amount of honey or maple syrup. However, keep in mind that added sugars should be limited on an RA diet.

3. To add more taste and nutrients, consider adding a pinch of cinnamon or ground ginger.

4. You can prepare a larger batch of porridge and store it in the refrigerator for up to 3 days.

NUTRITIONAL VALUES (PER SERVING):

Calories: 250 | Protein: 5 grams | Fat: 20 grams | Carbohydrates: 15 grams | Fiber: 10 grams

Serving Portion: 1 serving

Prep Time: 5 minutes

DIET RECIPE NOTES:

1. This recipe is generally suitable for an RA-friendly diet. It is rich in omega-3 fatty acids, fiber, and antioxidants, all of which have anti-inflammatory properties. The recipe is also naturally gluten-free and can be easily adapted to be vegan by using maple syrup instead of honey.

2. The amount of added sweetener should be limited or omitted altogether to align with the dietary recommendations for RA.

3. If you have any known sensitivities or allergies to the ingredients, please make appropriate substitutions.

_____

_____

_____

_____

_____

_____

3. Omelet with Spinach and Feta

A simple and nutritious breakfast or light lunch, this omelet is rich in anti-inflammatory ingredients. Eggs provide protein and healthy fats, while spinach offers vitamins and minerals. Feta cheese adds a tangy flavor and calcium. This recipe is quick and easy to prepare, making it a great option for busy mornings or when you're experiencing a flare-up.

INGREDIENTS:

- 2 large eggs

- 1/4 cup chopped fresh spinach

- 1/4 cup crumbled feta cheese

- 1 tablespoon olive oil

- Salt and pepper to taste

PREPARATION METHODS:

1. Mix eggs in a small bowl. Season with salt and pepper.

2. Heat olive oil in a small non-stick pan over medium heat.

3. Add spinach to the skillet and cook until wilted, about 1 minute.

4. Pour the egg mixture into the pan and let it cook for a few minutes until the edges start to set.

5. Sprinkle feta cheese over half of the omelet.

6. Carefully fold the omelet in half using a spatula.

7. Cook for another minute or until the cheese is melted and the omelet is cooked through.

8. Slide the omelet onto a plate and serve immediately.

PREP TIPS:

1. You can add other vegetables to this omelet, such as chopped mushrooms, bell peppers, or onions.

2. If you're sensitive to dairy, you can substitute the feta cheese with a plant-based option or omit it altogether.

3. To make this recipe even easier, you can pre-chop the spinach and crumble the feta cheese ahead of time.

NUTRITIONAL VALUES PER SERVING (1 OMELET):

Calories: 250 | Protein: 18g | Fat: 18g | Carbohydrates: 3g | Fiber: 1g | Sodium: 400mg (depending on the feta cheese) | Calcium: 150mg

Serving Portion: 1 omelet

Prep Time: 5 minutes

Cooking Time: 5-7 minutes

DIET RECIPE NOTE:

1. This recipe is suitable for an RA diet as it focuses on whole, unprocessed ingredients with anti-inflammatory properties.

2. Eggs are a good source of protein and healthy fats, while spinach provides vitamins, minerals, and antioxidants.

3. Feta cheese adds calcium, but if you are sensitive to dairy, you can substitute it with a plant-based cheese option or omit it altogether.

4. Olive oil is a healthy fat that can help reduce inflammation.

4. Mini Broccoli Frittatas

Mini Broccoli Frittatas are a nutritious and delicious breakfast option for individuals with rheumatoid arthritis. They are rich in anti-inflammatory ingredients like broccoli, eggs, and cheese, providing a good source of protein, vitamins, and minerals. Their convenient size makes them perfect for meal prep or a grab-and-go breakfast.

INGREDIENTS:

- 10 large eggs

- 1/2 cup milk (low-fat or non-fat)

- 1/2 teaspoon salt

- 1/4 teaspoon black pepper

- 1/4 teaspoon garlic powder

- 1/4 teaspoon onion powder

- 1 cup finely chopped broccoli florets

- 1/2 cup shredded cheddar cheese (low-fat or sharp)

PREPARATION METHOD:

1. Heat oven to 350°F (175°C). Grease a 12-cup muffin tin.

2. In a large bowl, mix eggs, milk, salt, pepper, garlic powder, and onion powder.

3. Stir in chopped broccoli and shredded cheese.

4. Divide the mixture evenly among the greased muffin cups.

5. Bake for 20-25 minutes, or until the frittatas are set and lightly golden on top.

6. Let cool in the muffin tin for a few minutes before removing and serving.

PREP TIPS:

1. You can option broccoli with other anti-inflammatory vegetables like spinach, kale, or bell peppers.

2. Use a combination of cheeses for added taste and variety.

3. For a dairy-free option, try using plant-based milk and cheese options.

4. Add a pinch of turmeric or other anti-inflammatory spices to the egg mixture.

5. Make a large batch ahead of time and store it in the refrigerator for a quick and easy breakfast throughout the week.

NUTRITIONAL VALUES PER SERVING (1 FRITTATA):

Calories: 120 | Protein: 10g | Fat: 8g | Carbohydrates: 3g | Fiber: 1g | Sodium: 200mg

Serving Portion: 2-3 frittatas

Prep Time: 15 minutes

Cooking Time: 20-25 minutes

DIET RECIPE NOTE:

1. This recipe is suitable for an RA-friendly diet as it focuses on whole, unprocessed ingredients with anti-inflammatory properties.

2. It is naturally gluten-free.

3. Use low-fat or non-fat dairy options to reduce saturated fat intake.

4. Be mindful of sodium content if you are monitoring your salt intake.

5. If nightshade vegetables are a trigger for your RA, avoid adding peppers or other nightshades to the recipe.

5. Egg Casserole with Sweet Potato and Kale

This delicious and nutritious egg casserole is a perfect breakfast or brunch option for individuals with rheumatoid arthritis. Rich in anti-inflammatory ingredients like sweet potatoes and kale, it provides a satisfying and energizing start to the day. The combination of protein from eggs, complex carbohydrates from sweet potatoes, and vitamins and minerals from kale makes it a well-balanced meal that supports overall health and well-being.

INGREDIENTS:

- 1 tablespoon olive oil

- 1 medium sweet potato, peeled and diced

- 1 small onion, chopped

- 2 cups kale, chopped

- 6 large eggs

- 1/2 cup milk (dairy or plant-based)

- 1/4 cup grated Parmesan cheese

- 1/4 teaspoon salt

- 1/8 teaspoon black pepper

PREPARATION METHODS:

1. Heat the oven to 350°F (175°C). Grease an 8x8-inch baking bowl with olive oil.

2. Heat the olive oil in a large pan over medium heat. Add the sweet potato and onion and cook, stirring occasionally, until softened, about 5-7 minutes.

3. Add the kale to the pan and cook until wilted, about 2-3 minutes.

4. In a medium bowl, mix the eggs, milk, Parmesan cheese, salt, and pepper.

5. Spread the sweet potato and kale mixture evenly in the prepared baking bowl. Pour the egg mixture over the vegetables.

6. Bake for 25-30 minutes, or until the casserole is set and lightly browned on top.

7. Let cool for a few minutes before serving.

PREP TIPS:

1. To save time, pre-chop the sweet potato, onion, and kale the night before.

2. You can use any type of milk you prefer, including almond milk, soy milk, or oat milk.

3. Feel free to add other vegetables to the casserole, such as mushrooms, bell peppers, or spinach.

4. For a spicier taste, add a pinch of red pepper flakes or cayenne pepper to the egg mixture.

NUTRITIONAL VALUES PER SERVING (ASSUMING 6 SERVINGS):

Calories: 200 | Protein: 12g | Carbohydrates: 18g | Fat: 10g | Fiber: 3g

Serving Portion: One square of the casserole

Prep Time: 15 minutes

Cooking Time: 25-30 minutes

DIET RECIPE NOTE:

1. This recipe is suitable for an RA-friendly diet. It is packed with anti-inflammatory ingredients, including sweet potatoes and kale.
2. The eggs provide a good source of protein, while the olive oil offers healthy fats.
3. This recipe is also gluten-free and can be easily adapted to be dairy-free by using plant-based milk and omitting the Parmesan cheese. If nightshades are a concern, omit the pepper.

_____

_____

_____

_____

_____

_____

6. Blueberry Oatmeal Bowl

A comforting and nutritious breakfast, the Blueberry Oatmeal Bowl is a fantastic way to start your day while adhering to an RA-friendly diet. Oats are a great source of fiber, which helps regulate digestion and may aid in reducing inflammation. Blueberries, rich in antioxidants, combat free radicals and contribute to overall health. This simple yet satisfying bowl is selected with various toppings to suit individual liking and dietary needs.

INGREDIENTS:

- 1/2 cup rolled oats (old-fashioned or quick-cooking)

- 1 cup milk (dairy or plant-based, unsweetened)

- 1/2 cup fresh or frozen blueberries

- 1/4 teaspoon ground cinnamon

- 1 tablespoon maple syrup or honey (optional)

- Optional toppings: chopped nuts, seeds, nut butter, yogurt, additional fruit

PREPARATION METHODS:

1. In a small saucepan, combine oats, milk, and blueberries.

2. Bring the mixture to a boil over medium heat, then reduce heat to low and cook for 5-7 minutes, or until the oats are cooked and the mixture has thickened.

3. Stir in cinnamon and sweetener (if using).

4. Transfer the oatmeal to a bowl and top with your desired toppings.

PREP TIPS:

1. For a creamier texture, use milk with a higher fat content or add a dollop of yogurt.

2. If using frozen blueberries, no need to thaw them before adding them to the pot.

3. Try different toppings, such as chopped nuts, seeds, nut butter, or additional fruit.

4. To make this recipe ahead of time, cook the oatmeal and store it in the refrigerator. Reheat it in the microwave or on the stovetop when ready to eat.

NUTRITIONAL VALUES PER SERVING:

Calories: 250-300 (depending on toppings) | Protein: 8g | Carbohydrates: 40g | Fat: 5g | Fiber: 5g

Serving Portion: 1 bowl

Prep Time: 5 minutes

Cooking Time: 5-7 minutes

DIET RECIPE NOTE:

1. This recipe is highly suitable for an RA-friendly diet. It is naturally low in saturated and trans fats and can be easily adapted to be gluten-free by using certified gluten-free oats. It is also free of nightshade vegetables.
2. The sweetness can be adjusted or completely omitted to cater to individual likeness or dietary limitations. If choosing dairy milk, option for low-fat or skim varieties.

Additional Notes for RA Considerations:

1. While generally healthy, some individuals with RA may find nuts and seeds aggravate their symptoms. If this is the case, consider omitting them or trying options like ground flaxseed or hemp seeds.

2. If you're sensitive to added sugars, feel free to omit the maple syrup or honey, or use a natural, zero-calorie sweetener like stevia.

3. If you have lactose intolerance or suspect dairy triggers your RA symptoms, use a plant-based milk option such as almond milk, oat milk, or soy milk.

7. Sweet Potato–Ground Turkey Hash

This delicious and nutritious hash is a fantastic option for those following an anti-inflammatory diet for rheumatoid arthritis. Sweet potatoes, rich in antioxidants and fiber, provide sustained energy and help regulate blood sugar levels. Ground turkey offers lean protein, essential for muscle maintenance and repair. The addition of herbs and spices helps taste while potentially offering additional anti-inflammatory benefits.

INGREDIENTS:

- 1 tablespoon olive oil

- 1 pound ground turkey

- 1 medium sweet potato, peeled and diced

- 1/2 onion, chopped

- 1 bell pepper (any color), chopped (optional, check for nightshade sensitivity)

- 1/2 teaspoon dried thyme

- 1/4 teaspoon salt

- 1/8 teaspoon black pepper

PREPARATION METHOD:

1. Heat the olive oil in a large pan over medium heat. Add the ground turkey and cook, breaking it up with a spoon, until browned.

2. Add the sweet potato, onion, and bell pepper (if using) to the pan. Cook, stirring occasionally, until the vegetables are softened, about 10-12 minutes.

3. Stir in the thyme, salt, and pepper. Cook for 1-2 minutes more, or until heated through.

4. Serve hot, garnished with fresh herbs, if desired.

PREP TIPS:

1. To save time, pre-chop the sweet potato, onion, and bell pepper ahead of time.

2. You can use any type of ground meat you like, such as chicken or beef. However, opt for leaner varieties to reduce saturated fat intake.

3. Feel free to try with different herbs and spices, such as rosemary, sage, or paprika.

4. For a boost of taste, add a squeeze of lemon juice or a sprinkle of balsamic vinegar just before serving.

NUTRITIONAL VALUES PER SERVING (ASSUMING 4 SERVINGS):

Calories: 300 | Protein: 25g | Carbohydrates: 25g | Fat: 12g | Fiber: 4g

Serving Portion: 1/4 of the recipe

Prep Time: 10 minutes

Cooking Time: 15-20 minutes

DIET RECIPE NOTE:

This recipe is generally suitable for an RA-friendly diet. It features anti-inflammatory ingredients like sweet potatoes and incorporates lean protein. The use of olive oil provides healthy fats.

Considerations:

1. If you're sensitive to nightshades, omit the bell pepper or substitute it with another vegetable like zucchini or mushrooms.

2. Adjust the amount of black pepper or other spices to your choice.

3. Be mindful of the sodium content if you're monitoring your intake. You can adjust the amount of salt or use a low-sodium broth if needed.

8. Overnight "Porridge" with Banana

This simple and satisfying overnight "porridge" is a great make-ahead breakfast for those with rheumatoid arthritis. The combination of rolled oats, banana, and milk creates a creamy and nutritious meal that's gentle on the digestive system and rich in anti-inflammatory benefits. The addition of chia seeds boosts the fiber and omega-3 content, while a touch of cinnamon adds warmth and taste.

INGREDIENTS:

- 1/2 cup rolled oats

- 1/2 cup milk (dairy or plant-based, such as almond or oat milk)

- 1/2 mashed banana

- 1 tablespoon chia seeds

- 1/4 teaspoon ground cinnamon (optional)

- Optional toppings: berries, sliced banana, chopped nuts, seeds, a sprinkle of honey or maple syrup (use sparingly)

PREPARATION METHOD:

1. In a jar or bowl, combine the rolled oats, milk, mashed banana, chia seeds, and cinnamon (if using).

2. Stir well to combine all the ingredients.

3. Cover the jar or bowl and refrigerate overnight, or for at least 4 hours.

4. In the morning, give the porridge a quick stir. Add a splash of milk if it's too thick.

5. Top with your desired toppings and enjoy!

PREP TIPS:

1. For a creamier texture, use full-fat milk or yogurt instead of regular milk.

2. If you like a warmer breakfast, gently heat the porridge in a saucepan over low heat or the microwave for a few seconds.

3. Try with different toppings to add variety and additional nutrients.

NUTRITIONAL VALUES PER SERVING:

Calories: 250-300 (depending on toppings) | Protein: 8-10g | Carbohydrates: 35-40g | Fat: 10-12g | Fiber: 5-7g

Serving Portion: 1 serving

Prep Time: 5 minutes (overnight soaking)

DIET RECIPE NOTE:

1. A good source of fiber, which helps regulate digestion and may reduce inflammation

2. Rich in potassium and magnesium, which may help reduce inflammation and support muscle function

3. High in omega-3 fatty acids, known for their anti-inflammatory properties

4. May have anti-inflammatory and antioxidant effects

This recipe is naturally gluten-free if using great gluten-free oats. It can also be easily adapted to be vegan by using plant-based milk and omitting or substituting honey or maple syrup with a natural sweetener like stevia or monk fruit.

9. Almond Maple Muffins

These Almond Maple Muffins offer a delicious and nutritious way to start your day, especially if you're managing rheumatoid arthritis. The combination of almond flour, which is naturally gluten-free and low in inflammatory compounds, and the touch of sweetness from maple syrup makes them a satisfying and wholesome treat. These muffins are also rich in healthy fats and fiber, providing sustained energy and promoting gut health.

INGREDIENTS:

- 2 cups almond flour

- 1/2 cup tapioca flour (or arrowroot flour)

- 1 teaspoon baking powder

- 1/2 teaspoon baking soda

- 1/4 teaspoon salt

- 1/4 cup pure maple syrup

- 1/4 cup unsweetened applesauce

- 1/4 cup melted coconut oil

- 2 large eggs

- 1 teaspoon vanilla extract

- 1/2 cup chopped almonds (optional)

PREPARATION METHOD:

1. Heat oven to 350°F (175°C) and line a muffin tin with paper liners.

2. In a large bowl, mix the almond flour, tapioca flour, baking powder, baking soda, and salt.

3. In a separate bowl, mix the maple syrup, applesauce, melted coconut oil, eggs, and vanilla extract.

4. Pour the wet ingredients into the dry ingredients and stir until just combined. Do not overmix.

5. Fold in the chopped almonds (if using).

6. Divide the batter evenly among the prepared muffin cups.

7. Bake for 20-25 minutes, or until a toothpick inserted into the center comes out clean.

8. Let the muffins cool in the muffin tin for a few minutes before transferring them to a wire rack to cool completely.

PREP TIPS:

1. Make sure the coconut oil is completely melted and cooled slightly before adding it to the wet ingredients.

2. Do not overmix the batter, as this can result in tough muffins.

3. If you don't have tapioca flour, you can substitute it with arrowroot flour.

4. You can also add other mix-ins to the batter, such as blueberries, chopped walnuts, or shredded coconut.

NUTRITIONAL VALUES PER SERVING (ASSUMING 12 MUFFINS):

Calories: 180 | Protein: 5g | Carbohydrates: 15g | Fat: 13g | Fiber: 3g

Serving Portion: 1 muffin

Prep Time: 15 minutes

Cooking Time: 20-25 minutes

DIET RECIPE NOTE:

1. These Almond Maple Muffins are a great option for an RA-friendly diet.
2. They are made with anti-inflammatory ingredients like almond flour and maple syrup, and they are free of refined grains, added sugars, and unhealthy fats.
3. They are also gluten-free, making them suitable for individuals with gluten sensitivities or celiac disease.

10. Seeds and Fruit Granola

A hearty and wholesome breakfast or snack, this Seeds and Fruit Granola is rich in anti-inflammatory ingredients and provides sustained energy to make your day. The combination of nuts, seeds, and fruit offers a delicious mix of textures and taste, while the absence of refined sugars and processed ingredients makes it a great choice for individuals with RA.

INGREDIENTS:

- 3 cups rolled oats (gluten-free if needed)

- 1 cup mixed nuts (almonds, walnuts, pecans)

- 1/2 cup pumpkin seeds

- 1/2 cup sunflower seeds

- 1/4 cup chia seeds

- 1/4 cup flaxseeds

- 1/4 cup unsweetened shredded coconut

- 1/4 cup dried cranberries or cherries (unsweetened)

- 1/4 cup chopped dates or raisins

- 1/4 cup maple syrup or honey

- 1/4 cup melted coconut oil or olive oil

- 1 teaspoon vanilla extract

- 1/2 teaspoon ground cinnamon

- Pinch of sea salt

PREPARATION METHODS:

1. Heat oven to 300°F (150°C) and line a baking sheet with parchment paper.

2. In a large bowl, combine oats, nuts, seeds, coconut, and dried fruit.

3. In a separate small bowl, mix maple syrup (or honey), oil, vanilla extract, cinnamon, and salt.

4. Pour the wet ingredients over the dry ingredients and mix well until everything is evenly coated.

5. Spread the mixture onto the prepared baking sheet in a single layer.

6. Bake for 20-25 minutes, stirring every 10 minutes, until golden brown and until aroma comes out.

7. Let cool completely on the baking sheet before storing in an airtight container.

PREP TIPS:

1. You can make this recipe by using your favorite nuts, seeds, and dried fruits.

2. To make it nut-free, substitute the mixed nuts with additional seeds or oats.

3. For a lower-sugar option, omit the dried fruit or use a smaller amount.

4. Store the granola in an airtight container at room temperature for up to 2 weeks.

NUTRITIONAL VALUES PER SERVING (APPROXIMATELY 1/2 CUP):

Calories: 250-300 (depending on ingredients) | Protein: 7-10g | Carbohydrates: 30-40g | Fat: 10-15g | Fiber: 5-7g

Serving Portion: 1/2 cup

Prep Time: 10 minutes

Cooking Time: 20-25 minutes

DIET RECIPE NOTE:

1. This recipe is suitable for an RA-friendly diet as it is best for whole grains, nuts, seeds, and fruit, which are all rich in anti-inflammatory nutrients.

2. It's also free of refined sugars and processed ingredients. Remember to choose unsweetened dried fruits and avoid any nuts or seeds that you may be allergic to. If gluten is a concern, ensure you use gluten-free oats.

11. Quinoa Breakfast Bowl

A Quinoa Breakfast Bowl is a delicious and nutritious option that's perfect for people with rheumatoid arthritis. Quinoa, a complete protein rich in fiber and antioxidants, provides sustained energy and helps manage inflammation. This bowl can be made for with various toppings, making it a delicious and adaptable way to start your day.

INGREDIENTS:

- 1/2 cup cooked quinoa
- 1/2 cup unsweetened almond milk (or other preferred milk)
- 1/2 teaspoon cinnamon
- 1/4 teaspoon vanilla extract
- Pinch of salt (optional)

- Fresh or frozen berries (strawberries, blueberries, raspberries)
- Sliced banana
- Chopped nuts (almonds, walnuts)
- Seeds (chia, flax, pumpkin)
- Unsweetened coconut flakes
- Sprinkle of honey or maple syrup (optional)

TOPPINGS:

PREPARATION METHODS:

1. If using uncooked quinoa, rinse thoroughly and cook according to package instructions.

2. In a small saucepan, combine the cooked quinoa, almond milk, cinnamon, vanilla extract, and salt (if using).

3. Heat over medium heat, stirring occasionally, until warmed through.

4. Pour the quinoa mixture into a bowl and top with your desired toppings.

5. Enjoy warm!

PREP TIPS:

1. Cook a larger batch of quinoa in advance to have on hand for quick breakfasts throughout the week.

2. Try with different toppings to find your favorite combinations.

3. For a creamier texture, use full-fat coconut milk instead of almond milk.

4. Add a pinch of turmeric or ginger for additional anti-inflammatory benefits.

NUTRITIONAL VALUES PER SERVING (WILL VARY BASED ON TOPPINGS):

Calories: 250-350 | Protein: 8-12g | Carbohydrates: 30-40g | Fat: 10-15g | Fiber: 5-7g

Serving Portion: 1 bowl

Prep Time: 5 minutes

Cooking Time: 5-10 minutes (if using pre-cooked quinoa)

DIET RECIPE NOTE:

1. This recipe is highly suitable for an RA-friendly diet. Quinoa is a gluten-free whole grain rich in protein, fiber, and antioxidants.
2. The addition of fruits, nuts, and seeds further boosts the anti-inflammatory benefits. Be mindful of added sugars by using unsweetened milk and limiting or omitting sweeteners like honey or maple syrup.

_____

_____

_____

_____

_____

_____

_____

_____

12. Lemon Vanilla Pancakes

These fluffy and spicy pancakes offer a delicious way to start your day. The combination of bright lemon zest and warm vanilla extract creates a balanced sweetness that's both satisfying and refreshing. With a few simple adjustments, these pancakes can easily fit into an anti-inflammatory diet, making them a suitable choice for individuals with rheumatoid arthritis.

INGREDIENTS:

- 1 cup all-purpose flour (can substitute with a gluten-free blend if needed)

- 2 tablespoons coconut sugar (or another natural sweetener)

- 2 teaspoons baking powder

- 1/2 teaspoon baking soda

- 1/4 teaspoon salt

- 1 cup unsweetened almond milk (or other dairy-free milk)

- 1 tablespoon lemon zest

- 1 large egg

- 1 teaspoon vanilla extract

- 2 tablespoons melted coconut oil (or other healthy oil)

- Optional toppings: fresh berries, sliced bananas, chopped nuts, a drizzle of honey or maple syrup

PREPARATION METHODS:

1. In a large bowl, mix the flour, coconut sugar, baking powder, baking soda, and salt.

2. In a separate bowl, mix the almond milk, lemon zest, egg, and vanilla extract.

3. Add the wet ingredients to the dry ingredients and stir until just combined. Don't overmix; a few lumps are okay.

4. Gently fold in the melted coconut oil.

5. Heat a large pan or griddle over medium heat. Lightly grease with coconut oil or cooking spray.

6. Pour 1/4 cup of batter onto the hot pan for each pancake. Cook until bubbles form on the surface and the edges look set, then flip and cook until golden brown on the other side.

7. Serve warm with your desired toppings.

PREP TIPS:

1. For fluffier pancakes, let the batter rest for 5-10 minutes before cooking.

2. If the batter is too thick, add a tablespoon or two of additional milk.

3. To make ahead, cook the pancakes and store them in the refrigerator or freezer. Reheat in a toaster or oven when ready to serve.

NUTRITIONAL VALUES PER SERVING (ASSUMING 4 SERVINGS):

Calories: 250-300 (depending on toppings) | Protein: 8g | Carbohydrates: 35-40g | Fat: 10-12g | Fiber: 3-4g

Serving Portion: 2-3 pancakes

Prep Time: 10 minutes

Cooking Time: 15-20 minutes

DIET RECIPE NOTE:

1. The recipe calls for all-purpose flour, which is a refined grain. Consider substituting it with a gluten-free blend or a mix of whole-wheat and oat flour for added fiber and nutrients.

2. Coconut sugar is a less processed alternative to refined white sugar, but it's still a form of sugar. Use it in moderation or explore other natural sweeteners like honey or maple syrup.

3. Choose toppings wisely. Fresh berries and sliced bananas are excellent anti-inflammatory options. Limit added sugars from syrups or honey.

13. Spinach and Mushroom Frittata

Frittatas are delicious and nutritious meals that can be enjoyed for breakfast, lunch, or dinner. This Spinach and Mushroom Frittata is rich in anti-inflammatory ingredients and protein, making it a great option for individuals with Rheumatoid Arthritis.

INGREDIENTS:

- 8 large eggs

- 1/4 cup milk (low-fat or plant-based alternative)

- 1/2 cup grated Parmesan cheese (or a dairy-free alternative)

- 1/2 teaspoon salt

- 1/4 teaspoon black pepper

- 2 tablespoons olive oil

- 1 small onion, diced

- 8 oz mushrooms, sliced

- 2 cloves garlic, minced

- 5 oz fresh baby spinach

PREPARATION METHODS:

1. Heat oven to 350°F (175°C).

2. Mix eggs, milk, Parmesan cheese, salt, and pepper in a bowl.

3. Heat olive oil in an oven-safe pan over medium heat.

4. Add the onion and cook until softened, about 3-4 minutes.

5. Add mushrooms and cook until browned, about 5-6 minutes.

6. Stir in minced garlic and cook for another minute.

7. Add spinach and cook until wilted, about 2-3 minutes.

8. Pour the egg mixture over the vegetables in the pan.

9. Cook on the stovetop for a few minutes until the edges start to set.

10. Transfer the pan to the preheated oven and bake for 10-12 minutes or until the frittata is set and lightly golden on top.

PREP TIPS:

1. You can substitute the spinach with other leafy greens like kale or Swiss chard.

2. Feel free to add other vegetables or herbs to the frittata, such as bell peppers, zucchini, or fresh thyme.

3. For a dairy-free option, use a plant-based milk alternative and omit the Parmesan cheese or replace it with a dairy-free cheese alternative.

NUTRITIONAL VALUES PER SERVING (ASSUMING 6 SERVINGS):

Calories: 200-250 calories | Protein: 15-18g | Carbohydrates: 5-7g | Fat: 15-18g | Fiber: 2-3g

Serving Portion: One slice

Prep Time: 15 minutes

Cooking Time: 20-25 minutes

DIET RECIPE NOTE:

1. This Spinach and Mushroom Frittata is suitable for an RA-friendly diet. It is rich in anti-inflammatory ingredients like spinach and mushrooms and provides a good source of protein from eggs.

2. The use of olive oil adds healthy fats. This recipe is naturally gluten-free. If you need to avoid dairy, you can substitute the milk and cheese with dairy-free options.

14. Salmon and Vegetable Frittata

A frittata is a delicious and nutritious meal that can be enjoyed for breakfast, lunch, or dinner. This Salmon and Vegetable Frittata is a powerhouse of anti-inflammatory ingredients, making it a great choice for people with rheumatoid arthritis. The combination of omega-3-rich salmon, vitamin-packed vegetables, and protein from eggs creates a satisfying and balanced meal that can help manage inflammation and promote overall health.

INGREDIENTS:

- 1 tablespoon olive oil

- 1/2 cup chopped onion

- 1 cup chopped mixed vegetables (e.g., broccoli florets, bell peppers, zucchini)

- 4 ounces cooked salmon, flaked

- 6 large eggs

- 1/4 cup milk (dairy or plant-based)

- 1/4 cup grated Parmesan cheese (optional)

- Salt and pepper to taste

- Fresh herbs (e.g., dill, parsley) for garnish (optional)

PREPARATION METHODS:

1. Heat oven to 350°F (175°C).

2. Heat the olive oil in an oven-safe pan over medium heat.

3. Add the chopped onion and cook until softened about 5 minutes.

4. Add the mixed vegetables and cook until soft-crisp, about 5-7 minutes.

5. Stir in the flaked salmon.

6. In a separate bowl, mix the eggs, milk, Parmesan cheese (if using), salt, and pepper.

7. Pour the egg mixture over the vegetables and salmon in the pan.

8. Transfer the pan to the preheated oven and bake for 15-20 minutes, or until the frittata is set and lightly golden on top.

9. Garnish with fresh herbs (if using) and serve warm or at room temperature.

PREP TIPS

1. Use leftover cooked salmon or canned salmon for convenience

2. You can substitute any of your favorite vegetables for the mixed vegetables.

3. If you don't have an oven-safe pan, you can transfer the mixture to a greased baking bowl before baking.

4. Add a pinch of red pepper flakes for a little spice

NUTRITIONAL VALUES PER SERVING (ASSUMING 6 SERVINGS):

Calories: 250 | Protein: 20g | Carbohydrates: 10g | Fat: 15g | Fiber3g

Omega-3 fatty acids: significant amount from salmon

Serving Portion: 1/6 of the frittata

Prep Time: 15 minutes

Cooking Time: 20 minutes

DIET RECIPE NOTE:

1. Salmon is a nice source of omega-3 fatty acids, known for their anti-inflammatory properties.

2. The variety of vegetables adds vitamins, minerals, and antioxidants that support overall health and combat inflammation

3. Eggs and salmon provide a good source of protein, essential for building and repairing tissues.

4. Olive oil provides healthy fats, which are important for nutrient absorption and overall well-being.

15. Omelet with Spinach and Feta

A simple yet satisfying breakfast or light lunch, this omelet is rich in nutrients and flavor, making it a great choice for those managing rheumatoid arthritis. Eggs offer a good source of protein, while spinach gives essential vitamins and minerals, including anti-inflammatory compounds. Feta cheese adds a creamy texture and a tangy taste, and its relatively low lactose content makes it easier to digest for those with sensitivities.

INGREDIENTS:

- 2 large eggs

- 1 tablespoon milk (or unsweetened plant-based milk option)

- Salt and pepper to taste

- 1 teaspoon olive oil

- 1/2 cup fresh spinach leaves

- 1/4 cup crumbled feta cheese

PREPARATION METHODS:

1. In a small bowl, mix the eggs, milk, salt, and pepper.

2. Heat the olive oil in a small non-stick pan over medium heat.

3. Add the spinach leaves and cook until wilted, about 1 minute.

4. Pour the egg mixture into the pan and swirl to coat the bottom evenly.

5. As the omelet cooks, gently lift the edges with a spatula to allow the uncooked egg to flow underneath.

6. When the omelet is almost set, sprinkle the feta cheese over half of the omelet.

7. Using the spatula, carefully fold the omelet in half.

8. Cook for a few more seconds until the cheese is slightly melted.

9. Slide the omelet onto a plate and serve immediately.

PREP TIPS:

1. For a fluffier omelet, add a pinch of baking powder to the egg mixture.

2. You can substitute spinach with other leafy greens like kale or Swiss chard.

3. Try with different cheeses or add other vegetables like mushrooms or bell peppers.

4. If you prefer a vegan option, use a plant-based cheese alternative and substitute the eggs with a chickpea flour batter.

NUTRITIONAL VALUES PER SERVING:

Calories: 250 | Protein: 15g | Carbohydrates: 3g | Fat: 20g

Serving Portion: 1 omelet

Prep Time: 5 minutes **Cooking Time:** 5-7 minutes

DIET RECIPE NOTE:

1. This recipe is suitable for an RA-friendly diet. It focuses on whole, unprocessed ingredients and is low in added sugars and unhealthy fats.

2. The olive oil provides healthy fats, while the spinach and feta offer essential nutrients. Eggs are a good source of protein and vitamin D, both important for managing RA.

3. Feta cheese, being lower in lactose than other cheeses, may be tolerated better by those with sensitivities.

Self-Reflection Questions:

1. What are my current breakfast habits, and how do they affect my RA symptoms?

_____

_____

_____

_____

_____

_____

2. Which anti-inflammatory ingredients do I enjoy, and how can I incorporate them into my breakfasts more frequently?

_____

_____

_____

_____

_____

_____

3. What challenges do I face when preparing breakfast, and how can the recipes in this chapter address those challenges?

_____

_____

_____

_____

_____

_____

4. How can I make breakfast a more mindful and enjoyable experience, even when I feel unwell?

5. What are my goals for incorporating a more anti-inflammatory breakfast routine into my life, and how will I measure my progress?

_____

_____

_____

_____

_____

_____

Date: _____

Monday:_____

_____

_____

Tuesday:_____

_____

_____

Wednesday:_____

_____

_____

Thursday:_____

_____

_____

Friday:_____

_____

_____

Saturday:_____

_____

_____

Sunday:_____

_____

_____

Exercise/Observation:_____

_____

_____

_____

CHAPTER 4:
RA-FRIENDLY MEAL FOR LUNCH DIET

1. Herbed Lettuce Rolls with Peach Sauce

These Herbed Lettuce Rolls with Peach Sauce offer a refreshing and light lunch option that aligns perfectly with an RA-friendly diet. They are rich in good taste and textures, featuring crisp lettuce leaves filled with a zesty herb-infused filling and sprinkled with a sweet and tangy peach sauce. This meal is not only delicious but also boasts a wealth of nutrients and anti-inflammatory benefits, making it an ideal choice for individuals managing rheumatoid arthritis.

INGREDIENTS:

FOR THE FILLING:

- 1 cup cooked quinoa, cooled
- 1/2 cup chopped cucumber
- 1/4 cup chopped red onion
- 1/4 cup chopped fresh parsley
- 1/4 cup chopped fresh mint
- 1 tablespoon lemon juice
- 1 tablespoon olive oil

- Salt and pepper to taste
- Large lettuce leaves (butter lettuce or romaine work well)

FOR THE PEACH SAUCE:

- 1 ripe peach, pitted and chopped
- 1 tablespoon lemon juice
- 1 tablespoon olive oil
- Pinch of salt

PREPARATION METHODS:

1. combine the cooked quinoa, cucumber, red onion, parsley, mint, lemon juice, olive oil, salt, and pepper in a medium bowl. Mix well until all the ingredients are evenly distributed.

2. combine the chopped peach, lemon juice, olive oil, and salt in a blender or food processor. Blend until smooth and creamy.

3. Wash and dry the lettuce leaves. Spoon a generous amount of the filling into the center of each lettuce leaf. Roll up the leaves tightly, tucking in the sides to secure the filling.

4. Arrange the lettuce rolls on a plate and sprinkle with the peach sauce. Enjoy immediately.

PREP TIPS:

1. Cook the quinoa ahead of time to save on preparation time.

2. You can substitute quinoa with other grains like brown rice or millet.

3. Feel free to try different herbs and spices in the filling.

4. If peaches are not in season, you can use frozen peaches or substitute with another fruit like mango or pineapple.

5. To make this recipe vegan, use a plant-based yogurt option in the peach sauce.

NUTRITIONAL VALUES PER SERVING (2 LETTUCE ROLLS):

Calories: 250-300 (depending on the type of lettuce and filling amount) | Protein: 10-12g | Carbohydrates: 30-35g | Fat: 12-15g | Fiber: 5-7g

Serving Portion: 2 lettuce rolls

Prep Time: 20 minutes

Cooking Time: 10 minutes (for cooking the quinoa, if not already cooked)

DIET RECIPE NOTE:

1. This recipe is a great choice for an RA-friendly diet. It is rich in fresh vegetables, herbs, and fruit, providing a wealth of anti-inflammatory nutrients.
2. The quinoa offers a good source of protein and fiber, while the olive oil contributes healthy fats. This meal is naturally low in saturated and trans fats, added sugars, and sodium.
3. It is also gluten-free and can be easily adapted to be vegan.

2. Zucchini and Avocado with Coconut-Lime Dressing

This bright and refreshing salad is a delicious addition to any RA-friendly meal plan. The combination of zucchini and avocado offers a wealth of nutrients, including vitamins, minerals, and healthy fats, which are known to support joint health and combat inflammation. The creamy coconut-lime dressing adds a touch of tropical flair, while the fresh herbs help the overall flavor and nutritional profile of this meal.

INGREDIENTS:

FOR THE SALAD:

- 2 medium zucchinis, thinly sliced or spiralized

- 1 ripe avocado, diced

- 1/4 cup chopped fresh cilantro

- 1/4 cup chopped fresh mint

- 1/4 cup toasted coconut flakes (unsweetened)

FOR THE COCONUT-LIME DRESSING:

- 1/4 cup full-fat coconut milk

- 1 tablespoon lime juice

- 1 tablespoon olive oil

- 1 teaspoon honey (or maple syrup, if preferred)

- 1/2 teaspoon grated ginger

- Pinch of salt and pepper

PREPARATION METHODS:

1. In a small bowl, mix the coconut milk, lime juice, olive oil, honey (or maple syrup), ginger, salt, and pepper until well combined.

2. In a large bowl, gently toss together the zucchini, avocado, cilantro, and mint.

3. Sprinkle the coconut-lime dressing over the salad and sprinkle with toasted coconut flakes. Serve immediately or chill for later.

PREP TIPS:

1. For a more visually appealing presentation, use a spiralizer to create zucchini noodles.

2. To toast the coconut flakes, place them in a dry pan over medium heat and cook, stirring frequently, until golden brown and aroma is out.

3. If you like a thicker dressing, you can add a tablespoon of Greek yogurt or mashed avocado to the coconut-lime mixture.

4. Feel free to add other vegetables or fruits to the salad, such as bell peppers, cherry tomatoes, or mango chunks.

NUTRITIONAL VALUES PER SERVING (ASSUMING 4 SERVINGS):

Calories: 250 | Protein: 5g | Carbohydrates: 15g | Fat: 20g | Fiber: 5g

Serving Portion: 1/4 of the salad

Prep Time: 15 minutes

DIET RECIPE NOTE:

1. This recipe aligns greatly with an RA-friendly diet. It prioritizes fresh, whole ingredients and is naturally low in sodium and added sugars.

2. The zucchini and avocado provide essential vitamins, minerals, and healthy fats, which are known to have anti-inflammatory properties.

3. The coconut milk and olive oil offer additional healthy fats, while the herbs contribute antioxidants and other good compounds.

_____

_____

_____

_____

_____

3. Asparagus and Beet Greens with Sesame Dressing

This great and nutritious salad is a bright way to start anti-inflammatory vegetables and healthy fats into your RA-friendly diet. Asparagus, rich in vitamins and minerals, is known for its potential to reduce inflammation. Beet greens, often overlooked, are rich in antioxidants and fiber. The sesame dressing, made with heart-healthy sesame oil, adds a nutty taste and provides a boost of omega-3 fatty acids.

INGREDIENTS:

- 1 bunch asparagus, trimmed

- 1 bunch beet greens, washed and chopped

- 1 tablespoon toasted sesame seeds

FOR THE SESAME DRESSING:

- 2 tablespoons olive oil

- 1 tablespoon sesame oil

- 1 tablespoon rice vinegar

- 1 teaspoon soy sauce (or tamari for gluten-free)

- 1 teaspoon honey (or maple syrup)

- 1/2 teaspoon grated ginger

- Pinch of red pepper flakes (optional)

PREPARATION METHODS:

1. Bring a pot of salted water to a boil. Add the asparagus and cook for 2-3 minutes, or until crisp-soft. Drain and immediately rinse with cold water to stop the cooking process.

2. Mix all the dressing ingredients until well combined in a small bowl.

3. In a large bowl, combine the cooked asparagus, chopped beet greens, and toasted sesame seeds. Pour the dressing over the salad and toss to coat evenly.

4. Serve immediately or chill for later.

PREP TIPS:

1. To toast sesame seeds, heat them in a dry pan over medium heat for a few minutes until they turn golden brown and fragrant.

2. If you like a milder flavor, omit the red pepper flakes from the dressing.

3. You can substitute rice vinegar with apple cider vinegar or white wine vinegar.

4. Feel free to add other vegetables to the salad, such as sliced radishes or shredded carrots.

5. For a more substantial meal, add grilled chicken or fish to the salad.

NUTRITIONAL VALUES PER SERVING (ASSUMING 4 SERVINGS):

Calories: 150 | Protein: 5g | Carbohydrates: 10g | Fat: 12g | Fiber: 4g

Serving Portion: 1 1/2 - 2 cups

Prep Time: 15 minutes

Cooking Time: 2-3 minutes

DIET RECIPE NOTE:

1. This salad is a great choice for an RA-friendly diet. It features nutrient-rich vegetables, healthy fats from olive and sesame oil, and minimal added sugars.

2. Asparagus and beet greens offer anti-inflammatory benefits, while the sesame seeds provide additional nutrients and texture.

3. The dressing is made with wholesome ingredients and can be easily adjusted to your taste liking.

4. Cream of Watercress and Spinach Soup

This tasty and velvety soup is a nourishing delight, great for those seeking comfort and relief from rheumatoid arthritis symptoms. The combination of watercress and spinach, both rich in anti-inflammatory compounds and essential nutrients, creates a powerful elixir to support overall health. The creamy texture, achieved without the use of heavy cream, makes this soup both satisfying and gentle on the digestive system.

INGREDIENTS:

- 1 tablespoon olive oil

- 1 medium onion, chopped

- 2 cloves garlic, minced

- 4 cups vegetable broth

- 1 bunch watercress, roughly chopped

- 10 ounces fresh spinach

- 1/4 cup chopped fresh dill

- Salt and pepper to taste

- Optional: a dollop of plain Greek yogurt or a sprinkle of nutritional yeast for added creaminess and taste

PREPARATION METHODS:

1. Heat the olive oil in a large pot over medium heat.

2. Add the chopped onion and cook until softened and translucent, about 5 minutes.

3. Add the minced garlic and cook for an additional minute, until the aroma comes out.

4. Pour in the vegetable broth and bring to a boil.

5. Reduce heat to low, add the watercress, spinach, and dill.

6. Cook for 5-7 minutes, or until the greens are wilted and soft.

7. Remove from heat and let cool slightly.

8. Carefully transfer the soup to a blender and puree until smooth. (Be cautious when blending hot liquids!)

9. Season with salt and pepper to taste.

10. Return the soup to the pot and reheat gently if needed.

11. Serve warm with an optional dollop of Greek yogurt or a sprinkle of nutritional yeast.

PREP TIPS:

1. To save time, use pre-chopped onions and garlic.

2. If you like a thicker soup, cook it for a longer time to reduce the liquid or add a small potato, peeled and diced, along with the onion.

3. For a vegan option, omit the Greek yogurt and use a plant-based milk option or additional olive oil for creaminess.

NUTRITIONAL VALUES PER SERVING (ASSUMING 4 SERVINGS):

Calories: 150-200 (depending on added creaminess) | Protein: 5-7g | Carbohydrates: 15-20g | Fat: 10-12g | Fiber: 4-5g

Serving Portion: 1 1/2 - 2 cups

Prep Time: 10 minutes

Cooking Time: 15-20 minutes

DIET RECIPE NOTE:

1. This recipe aligns beautifully with an RA-friendly diet. It is abundant in leafy greens, known for their anti-inflammatory properties.

2. The use of olive oil provides healthy fats, while the vegetable broth keeps the soup light and hydrating. This recipe is naturally low in saturated and trans fats, added sugars, and sodium.

3. It is also gluten-free and can be easily adapted to be vegan.

5. Moroccan Parsnip Carrot Slaw

This tasty and spicy Moroccan Parsnip Carrot Slaw is a bright addition to any meal, offering a unique twist on the classic slaw. The combination of crunchy parsnips and carrots, along with aromatic spices like cumin and coriander, creates a tantalizing taste profile. This meal is not only delicious but also rich in nutrients and anti-inflammatory benefits, making it a perfect choice for individuals with rheumatoid arthritis.

INGREDIENTS:

- 3 cups shredded carrots

- 1 cup shredded parsnips

- 1/4 cup chopped fresh cilantro

- 1/4 cup chopped fresh parsley

- 1/4 cup sliced almonds, toasted

- 2 tablespoons olive oil

- 1 tablespoon lemon juice

- 1 teaspoon ground cumin

- 1/2 teaspoon ground coriander

- 1/4 teaspoon ground cinnamon

- Salt and pepper to taste

PREPARATION METHODS:

1. In a large bowl, combine the shredded carrots, parsnips, cilantro, and parsley.

2. In a small bowl, mix the olive oil, lemon juice, cumin, coriander, cinnamon, salt, and pepper.

3. Pour the dressing over the vegetables and toss to coat evenly.

4. Sprinkle with toasted almonds and serve immediately or chill for later.

PREP TIPS:

1. To toast the almonds, place them in a dry pan over medium heat and cook, stirring frequently, until aroma comes out and lightly browned.

2. You can use a food processor with a shredding attachment to quickly shred the carrots and parsnips.

3. For a spicier slaw, add a pinch of cayenne pepper or red pepper flakes to the dressing.

4. This slaw is deliciously served on its own, as a side meal, or as a topping for grilled chicken or fish.

NUTRITIONAL VALUES PER SERVING (APPROXIMATELY 1 CUP):

Calories: 200 | Protein: 4g | Carbohydrates: 25g | Fat: 12g | Fiber: 5g

Serving Portion: 1 cup

Prep Time: 15 minutes

Cooking Time: 5 minutes (to toast the almonds)

DIET RECIPE NOTE:

1. This Moroccan Parsnip Carrot Slaw is a great addition to an RA-friendly diet. It is loaded with vegetables, offering a wealth of vitamins, minerals, and antioxidants.

2. The olive oil provides healthy fats, while the spices like cumin and coriander have anti-inflammatory properties.

3. This meal is naturally low in saturated and trans fats, added sugars, and sodium, making it a nutritious and delicious choice for individuals managing rheumatoid arthritis.

6. Sweet Potato Sauerkraut Colcannon

Sweet Potato Sauerkraut Colcannon is a delicious twist on the local Irish meal, begin anti-inflammatory sweet potatoes and gut-friendly sauerkraut. This comforting and nourishing recipe is ideal for those with Rheumatoid Arthritis (RA) as it prioritizes whole foods and avoids ingredients known to exacerbate inflammation. The combination of sweet potatoes, leafy greens, and sauerkraut offers a blend of complex carbohydrates, vitamins, minerals, and probiotics, all of which support overall health and well-being.

INGREDIENTS:

- 2 pounds sweet potatoes, peeled and cubed

- 1 tablespoon olive oil

- 1 medium onion, chopped

- 2 cups chopped kale or cabbage

- 1 cup sauerkraut, drained and rinsed

- 1/4 cup milk (or unsweetened plant-based milk alternative)

- Salt and pepper to taste

PREPARATION METHODS:

1. Boil a pot of salted water. Add the cubed sweet potatoes and cook until soft, about 15-20 minutes. Drain well.

2. Heat the olive oil in a large pan over medium heat. Add the chopped onion and cook until softened about 5 minutes.

3. Add the chopped kale or cabbage and cook until wilted about 3-5 minutes.

4. Stir in the drained sauerkraut and cook for another minute.

5. Mash the cooked sweet potatoes with a potato masher or fork. Add the milk and season with salt and pepper to taste.

6. Gently fold the sautéed vegetables and sauerkraut into the mashed sweet potatoes until well combined.

7. Transfer the colcannon to a serving bowl and enjoy warm.

PREP TIPS:

1. To save time, you can roast the sweet potatoes instead of boiling them. Heat the oven to 400°F (200°C), toss the cubed sweet potatoes with olive oil, salt, and pepper, and roast for 20-25 minutes, or until soft.

2. Feel free to substitute kale with other leafy greens like spinach or Swiss chard.

3. If you like a creamier texture, add a bit more milk or a dollop of plain yogurt.

4. You can also add other spices like garlic powder, onion powder, or a pinch of nutmeg for additional taste.

NUTRITIONAL VALUES PER SERVING (ASSUMING 4 SERVINGS):

Calories: 250 | Protein: 5g | Carbohydrates: 45g | Fat: 8g | Fiber: 7g

Serving Portion: 1 cup

Prep Time: 15 minutes

Cooking Time: 25-30 minutes

DIET RECIPE NOTE:

1. This Sweet Potato Sauerkraut Colcannon is a fantastic option for individuals following an RA-friendly diet. It's rich in anti-inflammatory ingredients like sweet potatoes, kale (or cabbage), and sauerkraut.

2. The meal is also naturally low in saturated and trans fats and free of refined grains and added sugars.

3. The use of olive oil provides healthy fats, and the sauerkraut offers good probiotics that can support gut health, which is crucial for managing inflammation.

7. Kale and Pumpkin Seed–Stuffed Portobello Mushrooms

These Kale and Pumpkin Seed-Stuffed Portobello Mushrooms offer a delicious and nourishing vegetarian meal, perfect for those following an anti-inflammatory diet for rheumatoid arthritis (RA). Portobello mushrooms provide a hearty and tasty base, while the kale filling delivers a wealth of vitamins, minerals, and antioxidants. Pumpkin seeds add a satisfying crunch and a boost of healthy fats and protein. This meal is not only visually appealing but also incredibly satisfying, making it a great option for lunch or dinner.

INGREDIENTS:

- 4 large portobello mushrooms

- 1 tablespoon olive oil

- 1/2 teaspoon salt

- 1/4 teaspoon black pepper

- 1 bunch of kale, stems removed and chopped

- 1/4 cup chopped onion

- 2 cloves garlic, minced

- 1/4 cup toasted pumpkin seeds

- 1/4 cup crumbled feta cheese (optional)

PREPARATION METHODS:

1. Heat oven to 400°F (200°C).

2. Clean the portobello mushrooms: Remove the stems and gently scrape out the gills with a spoon.

3. Brush the mushrooms with olive oil and season with salt and pepper.

4. Place the mushrooms gill-side up on a baking sheet and roast for 10 minutes.

5. While the mushrooms are roasting, prepare the filling: Heat olive oil in a pan over medium heat. Add the onion and cook until softened about 5 minutes. Add garlic and cook for an additional minute, until the aroma comes out.

6. Add the chopped kale to the pan and cook until wilted about 3-5 minutes. Season with salt and pepper to taste.

7. Remove the mushrooms from the oven and fill each cap with the kale mixture.

8. Sprinkle with toasted pumpkin seeds and crumbled feta cheese (if using).

9. Return the mushrooms to the oven and bake for another 5-7 minutes, or until the filling is heated through and the cheese is melted (if using).

10. Serve immediately.

PREP TIPS:

1. To save time, you can buy pre-washed and chopped kale.

2. Toast the pumpkin seeds in a dry pan over medium heat until aroma and lightly browned.

3. If you like a vegan option, omit the feta cheese or use a plant-based cheese option.

4. You can add other vegetables to the filling, such as chopped bell peppers or zucchini.

NUTRITIONAL VALUES PER SERVING (1 STUFFED MUSHROOM):

Calories: 200-250 (depending on the size of the mushroom and added cheese) | Protein: 10-12g | Carbohydrates: 15-20 | Fat: 12-15 | Fiber: 5-7g

Serving Portion: 1 stuffed mushroom

Prep Time: 15 minutes

Cooking Time: 15-20 minutes

DIET RECIPE NOTE:

1. This recipe aligns well with an RA-friendly diet. It emphasizes whole, unprocessed ingredients and is naturally low in saturated and trans fats, added sugars, and sodium.

2. The portobello mushrooms, kale, and pumpkin seeds are packed with anti-inflammatory nutrients, including vitamins, minerals, and antioxidants. The olive oil provides healthy fats, while the optional feta cheese offers a source of protein and calcium.

8. Sweet Potatoes Stuffed with Lentils, Kale, and Sunflower Seeds

This hearty and nutritious meal combines the natural sweetness of sweet potatoes with the protein-rich lentils and the earthy taste of kale, creating a balanced and satisfying meal. It's a great option for those managing rheumatoid arthritis due to its abundance of anti-inflammatory ingredients and its ability to provide sustained energy and essential nutrients. The sunflower seeds add a delightful crunch and boost of healthy fats, further helping the nutritional value of this recipe.

INGREDIENTS:

- 2 medium sweet potatoes
- 1 cup cooked lentils
- 1 tablespoon olive oil
- 1/2 cup chopped onion
- 2 cloves garlic, minced
- 2 cups chopped kale
- 1/4 cup sunflower seeds
- Salt and pepper to taste

PREPARATION METHODS:

1. Heat oven to 400°F (200°C).

2. Scrub sweet potatoes and pierce them several times with a fork.

3. Bake the sweet potatoes for about 45-60 minutes, or until soft when pierced with a fork.

4. While the sweet potatoes are baking, heat the olive oil in a pan over medium heat. Add the onion and cook until softened about 5 minutes.

5. Add the garlic and cook for an additional minute, until the aroma comes out.

6. Stir in the kale and cook until wilted, about 2-3 minutes.

7. Add the cooked lentils to the pan and season with salt and pepper to taste. Cook for another minute or two to heat through.

8. Once the sweet potatoes are cooked, remove them from the oven and let cool slightly.

9. Cut a lengthwise slit in the top of each sweet potato and gently fluff the flesh with a fork.

10. Fill each sweet potato with the lentil and kale mixture.

11. Sprinkle with sunflower seeds and serve immediately.

PREP TIPS:

1. To save time, cook the lentils ahead of time or use canned lentils, rinsed and drained.

2. You can substitute kale with other leafy greens, such as spinach or Swiss chard.

3. For more taste, add a pinch of your favorite spices to the lentil and kale mixture, such as cumin, paprika, or chili powder.

4. Top with a dollop of plain Greek yogurt or a drizzle of tahini sauce for added richness and creaminess.

NUTRITIONAL VALUES PER SERVING (1 STUFFED SWEET POTATO):

Calories: 350-400 | Protein: 15-18g | Carbohydrates: 50-60g | Fat: 10-12g | Fiber: 10-12g

Serving Portion: 1 stuffed sweet potato

Prep Time: 15 minutes

Cooking Time: 45-60 minutes

DIET RECIPE NOTE:

1. This recipe aligns perfectly with an RA-friendly diet. It features nutrient-dense whole foods like sweet potatoes, lentils, and kale, all known for their anti-inflammatory properties.

2. The sunflower seeds provide healthy fats and additional protein. The recipe is naturally low in saturated and trans fats, added sugars, and sodium, making it a wholesome and satisfying option for managing RA.

9. Sautéed Kale with Garlic

Sautéed Kale with Garlic is a simple yet tasty side meal that perfectly complements various meals. It's a nutritional powerhouse, rich in vitamins, minerals, and antioxidants that can help fight inflammation and promote overall health. The quick cooking time and minimal ingredients make it a convenient and accessible option for individuals with RA, even on days when energy levels are low.

INGREDIENTS:

- 1 bunch of kale, stems removed and roughly chopped

- 2 tablespoons olive oil

- 3-4 cloves garlic, minced

- 1/4 teaspoon red pepper flakes (optional)

- Salt and pepper to taste

- 1 tablespoon lemon juice (optional)

PREPARATION METHODS:

1. Wash and thoroughly dry the kale leaves. Remove the tough stems and roughly chop the leaves.

2. Heat the olive oil in a large pan over medium heat.

3. Add the minced garlic and red pepper flakes (if using) to the pan and sauté until the aroma comes out, about 30 seconds. Be careful not to burn the garlic.

4. Add the chopped kale to the pan and toss to coat with the oil and garlic.

5. Season with salt and pepper to taste.

6. Cover the pan and cook for 3-5 minutes, or until the kale is wilted and tender but still retains some of its vibrant green color.

7. Stir in the lemon juice (if using) just before serving.

PREP TIPS:

1. To ensure the kale cooks evenly, make sure it's dry before adding it to the pan. Excess moisture can cause it to steam instead of sauté.

2. You can adjust the number of garlic and red pepper flakes to your liking.

3. If you don't have fresh garlic on hand, you can use garlic powder, but add it towards the end of cooking to prevent burning.

4. To add more depth of taste, consider adding a splash of vegetable broth or white wine to the pan along with the kale.

NUTRITIONAL VALUES PER SERVING (APPROXIMATELY 1 CUP COOKED):

Calories: 80-100 | Protein: 3-4g | Carbohydrates: 7-9g | Fat: 5-7g | Fiber: 2-3g | Vitamins and Minerals: Rich in Vitamin A, Vitamin C, Vitamin K, Calcium, and Potassium

Serving Portion: 1-2 cups (adjust based on individual needs and meal size)

Prep Time: 5 minutes

Cooking Time: 5-7 minutes

DIET RECIPE NOTE:

1. Kale is a nutritional powerhouse, rich in anti-inflammatory compounds and essential nutrients.

2. Olive oil provides healthy fats, which are beneficial for joint health and overall well-being.

3. Garlic has been locally used for its potential anti-inflammatory properties.

4. The recipe is naturally low in saturated and trans fats, added sugars, and sodium, making it a healthy choice for individuals with RA.

Considerations:

If nightshades are a concern, omit the red pepper flakes. Those watching their sodium intake should use salt sparingly. The recipe can be easily selected with additional herbs and spices, such as lemon zest, grated Parmesan cheese, or a sprinkle of balsamic vinegar.

10. Chicken Celeriac Chili

This Chicken Celeriac Chili offers a warm and comforting meal, ideal for those seeking an anti-inflammatory and nourishing option to support their RA management journey. Combining lean protein from chicken with the unique taste and potential anti-inflammatory benefits of celeriac, this dish is a satisfying and flavorful way to incorporate more vegetables into your diet. The blend of spices adds warmth and depth, while the inclusion of beans provides more fiber and protein.

INGREDIENTS:

- 1 tablespoon olive oil

- 1 pound boneless, skinless chicken breasts or thighs, cut into bite-sized pieces

- 1 medium onion, chopped

- 2 cloves garlic, minced

- 1 medium celeriac, peeled and diced

- 1 (14.5 ounces) can of diced tomatoes, undrained

- 1 (15 ounces) can of kidney beans, rinsed and drained

- 1 teaspoon chili powder

- 1/2 teaspoon ground cumin

- 1/4 teaspoon smoked paprika

- 1/4 teaspoon dried oregano

- Salt and pepper to taste

- Optional toppings: chopped cilantro, avocado slices, lime wedges

PREPARATION METHODS:

1. Heat the olive oil in a large pot or Dutch oven over medium heat.

2. Add the chicken pieces and cook until browned on all sides. Remove the chicken from the pot and set aside.

3. Add the onion and garlic to the pot and cook until softened about 5 minutes.

4. Add the diced celeriac, diced tomatoes, kidney beans, chili powder, cumin, smoked paprika, oregano, salt, and pepper to the pot. Stir to combine.

5. Return the chicken to the pot.

6. Bring the chili to a cook, then reduce heat to low and cook for 30-40 minutes, or

until the celeriac is soft and the taste has melded.

7. Serve hot, topped with your desired toppings.

PREP TIPS:

1. To save time, you can use pre-cooked chicken or rotisserie chicken.

2. If you like a spicier chili, add more chili powder or a pinch of cayenne pepper.

3. For a thicker chili, mash some of the beans against the side of the pot with a potato masher.

4. Feel free to add other vegetables to the chili, such as bell peppers, corn, or zucchini.

NUTRITIONAL VALUES PER SERVING (ASSUMING 6 SERVINGS):

Calories: 300-350 | Protein: 30-35g | Carbohydrates: 30-35g | Fat: 10-12g | Fiber: 10-12g

Serving Portion: 1 1/2 - 2 cups

Prep Time: 15 minutes

Cooking Time: 30-40 minutes

DIET RECIPE NOTE:

1. This Chicken Celeriac Chili is a suitable choice for an RA-friendly diet. It prioritizes whole, unprocessed ingredients and avoids added sugars, unhealthy fats, and excessive sodium.

2. The lean protein from chicken, along with the fiber and nutrients from celeriac and beans, makes this a filling and nourishing meal.

3. The spices offer potential anti-inflammatory benefits. Be sure to choose low-sodium canned tomatoes and beans or rinse them thoroughly to reduce sodium content.

11. Wild Rice Quinoa Salad with Grilled Vegetables and Feta

This spicy and tasty salad is a powerhouse of nutrients and anti-inflammatory ingredients, making it a great choice for individuals with rheumatoid arthritis. The combination of wild rice and quinoa provides a hearty base rich in fiber and protein, while the grilled vegetables add a smoky sweetness and an abundance of vitamins and minerals. The feta cheese lends a creamy, tangy touch, rounding out the taste and providing additional protein and calcium. This salad is not only delicious but also supports overall health and well-being, making it a perfect addition to an RA-friendly diet.

INGREDIENTS:

- 1/2 cup wild rice

- 1/2 cup quinoa

- 1 cup mixed grilled vegetables (such as zucchini, bell peppers, onions, and mushrooms)

- 1/2 cup crumbled feta cheese

- 1/4 cup chopped fresh herbs (such as parsley, mint, or dill)

- 1/4 cup extra virgin olive oil

- 2 tablespoons lemon juice

- Salt and pepper to taste

PREPARATION METHODS:

1. Cook the wild rice and quinoa according to package instructions. Fluff with a fork and set aside to cool.

2. Heat a grill or grill pan over medium heat. Toss the mixed vegetables with a sprinkle of olive oil, salt, and pepper. Grill the vegetables for a few minutes per side, or until soft and slightly charred.

3. In a large bowl, combine the cooked wild rice, quinoa, grilled vegetables, feta cheese, and chopped herbs.

4. In a small bowl, mix the olive oil, lemon juice, salt, and pepper.

5. Pour the dressing over the salad and toss gently to combine. Serve immediately or chill for later.

PREP TIPS:

1. You can grill the vegetables ahead of time and store them in the refrigerator for a quick and easy meal.

2. Feel free to make the vegetables based on your liking and seasonal availability.

3. To make this recipe vegan, omit the feta cheese or substitute it with a plant-based cheese option.

4. Add a pinch of red pepper flakes or a dash of hot sauce for a more kick of taste.

NUTRITIONAL VALUES PER SERVING (ASSUMING 4 SERVINGS):

Calories: 350-400 | Protein: 15-18g | Carbohydrates: 45-50g | Fat: 15-18g | Fiber: 5-7g

Serving Portion: 1 1/2 - 2 cups

Prep Time: 20 minutes

Cooking Time: 30-40 minutes (for cooking the grains and grilling the vegetables)

DIET RECIPE NOTE:

1. This recipe aligns well with an RA-friendly diet. It is rich in whole grains, vegetables, and healthy fats, providing vital nutrients and anti-inflammatory benefits.

2. The wild rice and quinoa offer a good source of fiber and protein, while the grilled vegetables contribute vitamins, minerals, and antioxidants.

3. The feta cheese adds a touch of creaminess and calcium. The olive oil used in the dressing provides heart-healthy fats and additional anti-inflammatory properties.

4. This salad is also naturally low in saturated and trans fats, added sugars, and sodium.

_____

_____

_____

_____

_____

12.   Grilled Eggplant and Zucchini Sandwiches

This simple yet satisfying sandwich is a delicious and nutritious option for those following an anti-inflammatory diet for managing rheumatoid arthritis. Grilling the eggplant and zucchini brings out their natural sweetness and adds a smoky char, while the addition of fresh herbs and a light spread helps the overall taste and texture. This recipe is a great way to incorporate more vegetables into your diet and enjoy a delicious, RA-friendly lunch or light dinner.

INGREDIENTS:

- 1 medium eggplant, sliced lengthwise about 1/2 inch thick

- 1 medium zucchini, sliced lengthwise about 1/4 inch thick

- 2 tablespoons olive oil

- 1 tablespoon balsamic vinegar

- Salt and freshly ground black pepper to taste

- 2 slices whole-grain bread

- 2 tablespoons hummus or other preferred spread (e.g., avocado mash, pesto)

- Fresh herbs (optional, such as basil, oregano, or thyme)

PREPARATION METHODS:

1. Heat your grill or grill pan to medium-high heat.

2. In a small bowl, mix the olive oil, balsamic vinegar, salt, and pepper.

3. Brush both sides of the eggplant and zucchini slices with the olive oil mixture.

4. Grill the eggplant and zucchini slices for about 2-3 minutes per side, or until soft and slightly charred.

5. While the vegetables are grilling, toast the bread slices lightly.

6. Spread each slice of bread with the hummus or your chosen spread.

7. Layer the grilled eggplant and zucchini slices on one slice of bread.

8. Add fresh herbs (if using) and top with the other slice of bread.

9. Cut the sandwich in half and serve immediately.

PREP TIPS:

1. For a vegan option, use a plant-based spread and ensure the bread is vegan-friendly.

2. You can add other grilled vegetables to the sandwich, such as bell peppers or mushrooms.

3. If you don't have a grill, you can cook the eggplant and zucchini in a grill pan or pan on the stovetop.

4. For a more intense taste, marinate the eggplant and zucchini in the olive oil mixture for 30 minutes to an hour before grilling.

NUTRITIONAL VALUES PER SERVING (1 SANDWICH):

Calories: 350-400 (depending on the type of bread and spread used) | Protein: 10-12g | Carbohydrates: 40-45g | Fat: 15-20g | Fiber: 5-7g

Serving Portion: 1 sandwich

Prep Time: 10 minutes

Cooking Time: 10-12 minutes

DIET RECIPE NOTE:

This recipe is well-suited for an RA-friendly diet. It prioritizes fresh vegetables and whole grains, which are rich in anti-inflammatory nutrients and fiber. The use of olive oil provides healthy fats, and grilling the vegetables adds flavor without the need for excessive oil or unhealthy cooking methods. This sandwich is naturally low in saturated and trans fats and can be easily adapted to be vegan or gluten-free.

13. Sweet Potato and Black Bean Enchiladas

These Sweet Potato and Black Bean Enchiladas present a delicious and nourishing meal that harmonizes perfectly with an anti-inflammatory diet, making them suitable for individuals managing rheumatoid arthritis. The meal combines the natural sweetness of sweet potatoes with the fiber and protein of black beans, all wrapped in a wholesome corn tortilla and baked to perfection with a tasty enchilada sauce. It's a hearty and comforting meal that provides essential nutrients without relying on inflammatory ingredients.

INGREDIENTS:

FILLING:

- 2 large sweet potatoes, peeled and cubed
- 1 tablespoon olive oil
- 1/2 onion, chopped
- 2 cloves garlic, minced
- 1 (15-ounce) can black beans, rinsed and drained
- 1 teaspoon chili powder
- 1/2 teaspoon cumin
- 1/4 teaspoon salt
- 1/4 teaspoon black pepper

OTHER:

- 8 corn tortillas
- 1 (15-ounce) can of enchilada sauce (ensure it's low in sodium and added sugar)
- 1/2 cup shredded cheddar cheese (optional)
- Fresh cilantro, for garnish (optional)

PREPARATION METHODS:

1. Heat oven to 400°F (200°C).

2. Toss sweet potatoes with olive oil, salt, and pepper. Spread on a baking sheet and roast for 20-25 minutes or until soft.

3. Meanwhile, sauté onion and garlic in a pan until softened.

4. In a large bowl, mash the roasted sweet potatoes. Add the sautéed onion and garlic, black beans, chili powder, cumin, salt, and pepper. Mix well.

5. Spread a thin layer of enchilada sauce in the bottom of a 9x13-inch baking bowl.

6. Warm the corn tortillas one at a time in a pan or microwave until pliable.

7. Spoon about 1/3 cup of the filling mixture onto each tortilla. Roll up tightly and place seam-side down in the baking bowl.

8. Pour the remaining enchilada sauce over the enchiladas.

9. Sprinkle with shredded cheese, if desired.

10. Bake for 15-20 minutes, or until the cheese is melted and bubbly.

11. Garnish with fresh cilantro, if desired.

PREP TIPS:

1. You can use canned sweet potatoes to save time, but make sure they are rich in water or juices, not syrup.

2. For a spicier option, add a pinch of cayenne pepper to the filling or use a hotter enchilada sauce.

3. To make this recipe vegan, omit the cheese or use a plant-based cheese option.

4. Leftover enchiladas can be stored in the refrigerator for up to 3 days.

NUTRITIONAL VALUES PER SERVING (ASSUMING 4 SERVINGS):

Calories: 400 | Protein: 15g | Carbohydrates: 55g | Fat: 15g | Fiber: 10g

Serving Portion: 2 enchiladas

Prep Time: 30 minutes

Cooking Time: 20-25 minutes

DIET RECIPE NOTE:

1. This recipe aligns well with an RA-friendly diet. It features whole, unprocessed ingredients like sweet potatoes, black beans, and corn tortillas. These provide complex carbohydrates, fiber, and plant-based protein, which are all important for managing inflammation.

2. The use of olive oil adds healthy fats, while spices like chili powder and cumin offer potential anti-inflammatory benefits. Be sure to choose a low-sodium enchilada sauce and limit or omit the cheese to keep sodium levels in check.

14. Broiled Salmon with Lemon and Herbs

This Broiled Salmon with Lemon and Herbs recipe offers a simple yet tasty way to enjoy the anti-inflammatory benefits of salmon. The omega-3 fatty acids found in salmon are known to help reduce inflammation and joint pain, making this meal a great addition to an RA-friendly diet. The bright taste of lemon and herbs complement the salmon beautifully, while the broiling method ensures quick cooking and easy cleanup.

INGREDIENTS:

- 4 salmon fillets (about 6 oz each)

- 1 tablespoon olive oil

- 1 lemon, zested and juiced

- 1 tablespoon chopped fresh dill

- 1 tablespoon chopped fresh parsley

- 1/2 teaspoon garlic powder

- 1/4 teaspoon salt

- 1/4 teaspoon black pepper

PREPARATION METHOD:

1. Heat the broiler.

2. Line a baking sheet with aluminum foil for easy cleanup.

3. Place the salmon fillets on the prepared baking sheet.

4. In a small bowl, mix the olive oil, lemon zest, lemon juice, dill, parsley, garlic powder, salt, and pepper.

5. Brush the salmon fillets with the herb mixture, making sure to coat them evenly.

6. Broil the salmon for 8-10 minutes, or until cooked through. The salmon should flake easily with a fork.

PREP TIPS:

1. For crispier skin, pat the salmon fillets dry with paper towels before brushing them with the herb mixture.

2. If you like a milder garlic flavor, use 1/4 teaspoon of garlic powder instead of 1/2 teaspoon.

3. You can substitute the fresh herbs with 1 teaspoon of dried dill and 1 teaspoon of dried parsley.

4. Serve the broiled salmon with a side of steamed vegetables or a salad for a complete meal.

NUTRITIONAL VALUES PER SERVING (1 SALMON FILLET):

Calories: 300 | Protein: 40g | Carbohydrates: 3g | Fat: 17g | Fiber: 0g

Serving Portion: 1 salmon fillet

Prep Time: 10 minutes

Cooking Time: 8-10 minutes

DIET RECIPE NOTE:

This recipe is **highly suitable** for an RA-friendly diet. Salmon is a fantastic source of omega-3 fatty acids, which have potent anti-inflammatory effects. The fresh herbs and lemon add a taste without relying on added sugars or unhealthy fats. Broiling is a healthy cooking method that doesn't require excessive oil. This meal is naturally gluten-free and low in sodium.

Additional Considerations:

1. Choose wild-caught salmon whenever possible, as it tends to be lower in contaminants than farmed salmon.

2. If you're watching your sodium intake, you can reduce the amount of salt in the recipe or omit it altogether.

3. Pair this salmon with a variety of colorful vegetables for a well-rounded, anti-inflammatory meal.

15. Chickpea and Spinach Quesadilla–Cauliflower Pilaf

This wholesome and satisfying meal pairs the protein-rich and delicious chickpea and spinach quesadilla with a light and nutritious cauliflower pilaf. It provides a balanced meal with a variety of textures and flavors, catering to an RA-friendly diet.

INGREDIENTS:

FOR THE QUESADILLA:

- 1 tablespoon olive oil
- 1/2 cup chopped onion
- 1 clove garlic, minced
- 1 (15 ounce) can chickpeas, drained and rinsed
- 1 cup fresh spinach leaves
- 1/4 cup crumbled feta cheese
- 1/4 teaspoon ground cumin
- 1/4 teaspoon chili powder

- Salt and pepper to taste
- 2 whole-wheat tortillas

FOR THE CAULIFLOWER PILAF:

- 1 head cauliflower, rice or finely chopped
- 1 tablespoon olive oil
- 1/4 cup chopped onion
- 1/4 cup chopped red bell pepper
- 1/4 cup chopped fresh parsley
- Salt and pepper to taste

PREPARATION METHODS:

1. Heat olive oil in a large pan over medium heat. Add onion and red bell pepper, and cook until softened about 5 minutes. Add the rice cauliflower, parsley, salt, and pepper. Cook, stirring occasionally, until the cauliflower is soft-crisp, about 5-7 minutes. Set aside.

2. In the same pan, heat olive oil over medium heat. Add onion and garlic, and cook until softened about 3 minutes. Add chickpeas, spinach, feta cheese, cumin, chili powder, salt, and pepper. Cook, stirring occasionally, until the spinach is wilted and the chickpeas are heated through about 5 minutes.

3. Place one tortilla on a clean work surface. Spoon half of the chickpea mixture onto one half of the tortilla. Fold the other half over the filling. Repeat with the remaining tortilla and filling.

4. Heat the same pan over medium heat. Cook each quesadilla for 2-3 minutes per side or until golden brown and the cheese is melted.

5. Cut each quesadilla into wedges and serve with the cauliflower pilaf.

PREP TIPS:

1. To save time, rice the cauliflower ahead of time or purchase pre-riced cauliflower.

2. You can use any type of cheese you like, or omit it for a vegan option.

3. Add other vegetables to the quesadilla filling, such as bell peppers or mushrooms.

4. Adjust the spices to your liking.

NUTRITIONAL VALUES PER SERVING (ASSUMING 2 SERVINGS):

Calories: 500-600 | Protein: 25-30g | Carbohydrates: 50-60g | Fat: 20-25g | Fiber: 10-12g

Serving Portion: 1 quesadilla and 1/2 of the cauliflower pilaf

Prep Time: 20 minutes

Cooking Time: 20 minutes

DIET RECIPE NOTE:

1. This recipe is suitable for an RA-friendly diet. It utilizes whole-wheat tortillas, a good source of fiber, and avoids refined grains.

2. The chickpeas and feta cheese offer protein, while the spinach and cauliflower give vital vitamins, minerals, and antioxidants. Olive oil is used for cooking, which is a healthy fat source.

3. This recipe is naturally low in saturated and trans fats and can be easily adapted to be vegan by omitting the cheese or using a plant-based option. If nightshades are a concern, simply leave out the bell pepper from the pilaf.

Self-Reflection Questions:

1. What are my current lunch habits, and how do they support or hinder my RA management?

_____
_____
_____
_____
_____
_____

2. Which anti-inflammatory ingredients do I enjoy in my lunches, and how can I explore new options to add variety and excitement?

_____
_____
_____
_____
_____
_____

3. What challenges do I face when preparing or accessing healthy lunches, and how can the recipes in this chapter offer solutions?

_____
_____
_____
_____
_____

4. How can I make lunchtime a more mindful and enjoyable experience, even on busy days?

_____
_____
_____
_____
_____
_____

5. What are my goals for incorporating more anti-inflammatory lunches into my routine, and how will I track my progress and celebrate my successes?

_____

_____

_____

_____

_____

_____

_____

_____

_____

_____

_____

_____

CHAPTER 5:
RA-FRIENDLY DISHES FOR DINNER DIET

1. Summer Fruit, Crab, and Arugula Salad with Mint Dressing

This tasty salad bursts with the fresh tastes of summer, combining sweet fruits, succulent crab meat, and peppery arugula. The mint dressing adds a refreshing touch, while the combination of textures and colors makes this meal as visually appealing as it is delicious. It's a light yet satisfying option that aligns perfectly with an RA-friendly diet, providing essential nutrients and anti-inflammatory benefits.

INGREDIENTS

FOR THE SALAD:

- 5 cups arugula, washed and dried

- 1 cup mixed summer fruits (sliced peaches, nectarines, plums, or berries)

- 1 cup cooked crab meat, shredded or flaked

- 1/4 cup toasted slivered almonds

- Optional: 1/4 cup crumbled feta cheese (omit for dairy-free)

FOR THE MINT DRESSING:

- 1/4 cup extra virgin olive oil

- 2 tablespoons lemon juice

- 1 tablespoon chopped fresh mint

- 1 teaspoon honey or maple syrup (adjust to taste)

- Salt and pepper to taste

PREPARATION METHODS:

1. In a small bowl, mix the olive oil, lemon juice, chopped mint, honey/maple syrup, salt, and pepper until well combined.

2. In a large bowl, combine the arugula, mixed fruits, crab meat, and toasted almonds.

3. Gently toss the salad with the mint dressing just before serving. Divide the salad among plates and optionally top with crumbled feta cheese.

PREP TIPS:

1. To toast the almonds, place them in a dry pan over medium heat and cook, stirring frequently, until aroma comes out and lightly browned.

2. Use ripe, seasonal fruits for the best taste.

3. If you don't have fresh mint, you can use 1/2 teaspoon of dried mint instead.

4. For a vegan option, omit the feta cheese and use maple syrup instead of honey in the dressing.

5. Feel free to add other anti-inflammatory ingredients to the salad, such as avocado slices or chopped walnuts.

NUTRITIONAL VALUES PER SERVING (ASSUMING 4 SERVINGS):

Calories: 350-400 (depending on the fruit and cheese used) | Protein: 20-25g | Carbohydrates: 25-30g | Fat: 20-25g | Fiber: 5-7g

Serving Portion: 1 large bowl

Prep Time: 15 minutes

Cooking Time: 5 minutes (for toasting the almonds)

DIET RECIPE NOTE:

1. This recipe aligns well with an RA-friendly diet. It features a variety of anti-inflammatory ingredients, including arugula, fruits, crab meat, and olive oil.

2. The crab gives lean protein and omega-3 fatty acids, while the fruits and vegetables offer essential vitamins, minerals, and antioxidants.

3. This salad is naturally low in sodium and added sugars, making it a healthy and satisfying meal option. If you're sensitive to dairy, simply omit the feta cheese.

2. Spinach Salad with Salmon and Avocado

This delicious and nutritious Spinach Salad with Salmon and Avocado is a delightful choice for individuals with rheumatoid arthritis. It combines the anti-inflammatory benefits of leafy greens, omega-3-rich salmon, and healthy fats from avocado, creating a satisfying and balanced meal that supports overall well-being. This salad is easy to prepare, visually appealing, and rich in taste and textures that will tantalize your taste buds.

INGREDIENTS:

FOR THE SALAD:

- 4 cups fresh baby spinach leaves

- 4 ounces cooked salmon, flaked or chopped

- 1 avocado, diced

- 1/4 cup red onion, thinly sliced

- 1/4 cup chopped walnuts or almonds

- Optional additions: cherry tomatoes, cucumber slices, pomegranate arils

FOR THE DRESSING:

- 2 tablespoons extra virgin olive oil

- 1 tablespoon lemon juice

- 1 teaspoon Dijon mustard

- 1/2 teaspoon honey (or maple syrup for a lower glycemic option)

- Salt and pepper to taste

PREPARATION METHODS:

1. In a small bowl, mix the olive oil, lemon juice, Dijon mustard, honey (or maple syrup), salt, and pepper until well combined.

2. In a large bowl, combine the spinach leaves, salmon, avocado, red onion, and walnuts (or almonds). Add any optional ingredients you desire.

3. Gently sprinkle the dressing over the salad and toss to coat evenly. Serve immediately and enjoy!

PREP TIPS:

1. To cook the salmon, you can bake, grill, or poach it. Make sure it is cooked through but still moist.

2. For a vegan option, substitute the salmon with smoked tofu or tempeh.

3. You can use any type of nuts or seeds you like, such as pecans, sunflower seeds, or pumpkin seeds.

4. If you are short on time, you can use pre-cooked salmon or canned salmon (make sure it is packed in water or olive oil, not oil).

5. To keep the avocado from browning, add it to the salad just before serving.

NUTRITIONAL VALUES PER SERVING:

Calories: 400-450 | Protein: 25-30g | Carbohydrates: 20-25g | Fat: 25-30g | Fiber: 5-7g

Serving Portion: 1 large bowl

Prep Time: 15 minutes

Cooking Time: 10-15 minutes (for cooking the salmon, if not already cooked)

DIET RECIPE NOTE:

1. This Spinach Salad with Salmon and Avocado is a great choice for individuals following an RA-friendly diet. It prioritizes whole, unprocessed ingredients and emphasizes anti-inflammatory components.

2. The spinach provides essential vitamins, minerals, and antioxidants, while the salmon offers a good source of omega-3 fatty acids, known for their anti-inflammatory properties. The avocado adds healthy fats, which support overall health and can help reduce inflammation.

3. The dressing is made with extra virgin olive oil, another source of healthy fats with anti-inflammatory benefits. The addition of lemon juice provides vitamin C and helps the taste, while

4. Dijon mustard adds a touch of tanginess. If you are watching your sugar intake, you can omit the honey or maple syrup or use a natural sweetener like stevia.

3. Coconut and Saffron Mussel Soup

This aromatic and spicy Coconut and Saffron Mussel Soup gives a delicious and nourishing dinner option for individuals with rheumatoid arthritis. The combination of mussels, rich in anti-inflammatory omega-3 fatty acids, and the subtle warmth of saffron creates a comforting and satisfying meal. The creamy coconut milk base adds a touch of richness without relying on heavy cream, making it a lighter and healthier choice.

INGREDIENTS:

- 2 pounds fresh mussels, scrubbed and debearded
- 1 tablespoon olive oil
- 1 small onion, chopped
- 2 cloves garlic, minced
- 1-inch piece ginger, peeled and grated
- 1/2 teaspoon ground turmeric
- Pinch of saffron threads
- 1/2 cup dry white wine
- 1 (13.5-ounce) can full-fat coconut milk
- 1/2 cup vegetable broth or water
- Salt and pepper to taste
- Chopped fresh cilantro for garnish

PREPARATION METHODS:

1. Heat the olive oil in a large pot over medium heat. Add the onion and cook until softened about 5 minutes.

2. Add the garlic, ginger, turmeric, and saffron to the pot and cook for 1 minute more, stirring constantly.

3. Pour in the white wine and bring to a simmer. Cook for 2-3 minutes, or until the alcohol has evaporated.

4. Add the coconut milk, vegetable broth (or water), and mussels to the pot. Cover and cook for 5-7 minutes, or until the mussels open. Discard any mussels that do not open.

5. Season with salt and pepper to taste.

6. Ladle the soup into bowls and garnish with chopped cilantro. Serve immediately with crusty bread, if desired.

PREP TIPS:

1. Soak the mussels in cold water for 20 minutes before cooking to help them release any sand or grit.

2. Scrub the mussels thoroughly with a brush to remove any barnacles or other debris.

3. Discard any mussels that are cracked or open before cooking.

4. You can adjust the amount of saffron to your liking. A little goes a long way, so start with a pinch and add more if desired.

5. For a spicier soup, add a pinch of red pepper flakes or chopped chili pepper to the pot along with the onion and garlic.

NUTRITIONAL VALUES PER SERVING (ASSUMING 4 SERVINGS):

Calories: 350 | Protein: 30g | Carbohydrates: 20g | Fat: 20g | Fiber: 3g

Serving Portion: 1 bowl of soup

Prep Time: 15 minutes

Cooking Time: 15-20 minutes

DIET RECIPE NOTE:

1. This recipe is suitable for an RA-friendly diet. Mussels are a great source of omega-3 fatty acids, which have anti-inflammatory properties.
2. The addition of turmeric and ginger further helps the anti-inflammatory benefits of this meal. Coconut milk provides healthy fats and a creamy texture without relying on heavy cream.
3. This soup is also naturally low in added sugars and can be easily adjusted to be low in sodium by using low-sodium broth or water and adjusting the amount of salt added.

4. Spicy Shrimp Veggie Noodle Soup

This Spicy Shrimp Veggie Noodle Soup is a delicious and nutritious meal that can be a comforting and nourishing option for people with rheumatoid arthritis. It combines lean protein from shrimp with a variety of colorful vegetables and a touch of spice, creating a satisfying and anti-inflammatory meal. The broth-based nature of this soup makes it easy to digest, while the abundance of vegetables provides essential vitamins, minerals, and antioxidants.

INGREDIENTS:

- 1 tablespoon olive oil
- 1 small onion, chopped
- 2 cloves garlic, minced
- 1 inch piece of ginger, peeled and grated
- 1 red bell pepper, thinly sliced
- 1 cup sliced mushrooms
- 1 cup broccoli florets
- 1/2 cup chopped carrots
- 1/4 teaspoon red pepper flakes (adjust to taste)
- 4 cups vegetable broth
- 1 pound peeled and deveined shrimp
- 4 ounces rice noodles (or your preferred gluten-free noodles)
- 1 tablespoon soy sauce (or tamari for gluten-free)
- 1 tablespoon lime juice
- Fresh cilantro, for garnish

PREPARATION METHODS:

1. Heat the olive oil in a large pot over medium heat. Add the onion and cook until softened about 5 minutes.

2. Add the garlic, ginger, bell pepper, mushrooms, broccoli, and carrots. Cook, stirring occasionally, until the vegetables are crisp-soft, about 5 minutes.

3. Stir in the red pepper flakes and cook for 30 seconds more.

4. Pour in the vegetable broth and bring to a boil. Reduce heat to medium-low, cover, and cook for 5 minutes.

5. Add the shrimp and noodles to the pot. Cook until the shrimp are pink and

cooked through and the noodles are soft about 3-5 minutes.

6. Stir in the soy sauce and lime juice.

7. Ladle the soup into bowls, garnish with fresh cilantro, and serve hot.

PREP TIPS:

1. To save time, chop the vegetables ahead of time.

2. You can use any type of vegetable you like in this soup.

3. If you don't have rice noodles, you can use other gluten-free noodles or even zucchini noodles.

4. Adjust the amount of red pepper flakes to your desired level of spice.

5. For a vegan option, substitute the shrimp with firm tofu or chickpeas.

NUTRITIONAL VALUES PER SERVING (ASSUMING 4 SERVINGS):

Calories: 300-350 | Protein: 25-30g | Carbohydrates: 30-35g | Fat: 10-12g | Fiber: 4-5g

Serving Portion: 1 bowl

Prep Time: 15 minutes

Cooking Time: 20-25 minutes

DIET RECIPE NOTE:

1. This Spicy Shrimp Veggie Noodle Soup is a suitable option for an RA-friendly diet. It is rich in anti-inflammatory ingredients like vegetables and spices.

2. The shrimp provides lean protein, while the rice noodles offer a source of carbohydrates. The use of olive oil adds healthy fats, and the broth base makes it easy to digest.

3. The recipe can be adjusted to individual likeness by varying the vegetables or spice level.

5. Shrimp Pad Thai

Shrimp Pad Thai is a delicious and nutritious meal that can be adapted to fit an anti-inflammatory diet for individuals with rheumatoid arthritis. This popular Thai noodle meal typically features rice noodles stir-fried with shrimp, eggs, vegetables, and a tangy sauce. By making a few mindful substitutions and adjustments, you can create an option that's both delicious and supportive of your health goals.

INGREDIENTS:

FOR THE PAD THAI:

- 8 oz wide rice noodles (look for brown rice noodles for a healthier option)

- 1 tbsp olive oil

- 1 lb. peeled and deveined shrimp

- 2 cloves garlic, minced

- 1 small red bell pepper, thinly sliced

- 1 cup bean sprouts

- 3 scallions, chopped

- 2 large eggs, lightly beaten

- Chopped cilantro, for garnish

- Lime wedges, for serving

FOR THE PAD THAI SAUCE:

- 3 tbsp fish sauce

- 2 tbsp tamarind paste

- 1 tbsp honey or maple syrup (adjust to taste)

- 1 tbsp rice vinegar

- 1 tsp chili garlic sauce (adjust to taste)

PREPARATION METHODS:

1. Cook the rice noodles according to package instructions. Drain and rinse with cold water to prevent sticking.

2. In a small bowl, mix all the sauce ingredients until well combined.

3. Heat the olive oil in a large wok or pan over medium-high heat. Add the shrimp and cook until pink and cooked through, about 2-3 minutes per side. Remove the shrimp from the pan and set aside.

4. Add the garlic and red bell pepper to the pan and stir-fry for 1-2 minutes until slightly softened. Push the vegetables to one side of the pan and add the beaten

eggs. Scramble the eggs until cooked through.

5. Add the cooked noodles, shrimp, bean sprouts, and sauce to the pan. Toss everything together until well coated and heated through.

6. Garnish with chopped scallions and cilantro. Serve immediately with lime wedges.

PREP TIPS:

1. Have all your vegetables chopped and sauce prepared before you start cooking for a smooth and efficient process.

2. If you can't find brown rice noodles, use another gluten-free noodle option or zucchini noodles for a lower-carb option.

3. Adjust the amount of chili garlic sauce to your desired level of heat.

4. Feel free to add other vegetables to the stir-fry, such as broccoli florets, snap peas, or shredded carrots.

5. If you like, you can substitute the shrimp with firm tofu or chicken.

NUTRITIONAL VALUES PER SERVING (ASSUMING 4 SERVINGS):

Calories: 400-450 | Protein: 30-35g | Carbohydrates: 40-45g | Fat: 15-20g

Serving Portion: 1 1/2 - 2 cups

Prep Time: 20 minutes

Cooking Time: 15-20 minutes

DIET RECIPE NOTE:

1. Adjust the amount of honey or maple syrup in the sauce or use a natural sweetener like stevia.

2. Use olive oil or avocado oil for stir-frying instead of oils high in omega-6 fatty acids.

3. Fish sauce can be high in sodium. Look for a low-sodium option or use less.

4. If you are sensitive to nightshades, omit the red bell pepper or substitute it with another vegetable.

6. Shrimp and Asparagus Skillet

This quick and easy pan meal combines succulent shrimp with crisp-soft asparagus, creating a delicious and nutritious meal that's perfect for those managing rheumatoid arthritis. Shrimp is a lean protein source rich in omega-3 fatty acids, while asparagus offers a wealth of vitamins, minerals, and antioxidants. The simple preparation and minimal ingredients make this recipe ideal for busy weeknights or when you're feeling less energetic.

INGREDIENTS

- 1 pound large shrimp, peeled and deveined

- 1 pound asparagus, trimmed and cut into 2-inch pieces

- 2 tablespoons olive oil

- 3 cloves garlic, minced

- 1/4 cup lemon juice

- 1/4 teaspoon salt

- 1/4 teaspoon black pepper

- Optional: Red pepper flakes for a touch of heat

- Fresh parsley for garnish

PREPARATION METHODS:

1. Pat the shrimp dry with paper towels. Season with salt and pepper.

2. Heat 1 tablespoon of olive oil in a large pan over medium-high heat. Add the shrimp and cook for 2-3 minutes per side, or until pink and cooked through. Remove the shrimp from the pan and set aside.

3. Add the remaining olive oil to the pan. Add the asparagus and cook, stirring occasionally, until crisp-soft, about 3-5 minutes.

4. Add the garlic to the pan and cook until the aroma comes out about 30 seconds.

5. Return the shrimp to the pan. Add the lemon juice and toss to combine. Cook

for an additional minute, or until heated through.

6. Season with additional salt and pepper to taste. Garnish with fresh parsley and serve immediately.

PREP TIPS:

1. You can use fresh or frozen shrimp for this recipe. If using frozen, make sure to thaw them completely before cooking.

2. To add more taste, marinate the shrimp in lemon juice and herbs for 30 minutes before cooking.

3. Feel free to add other vegetables to the pan, such as cherry tomatoes or sliced mushrooms.

4. Serve this meal over brown rice or quinoa for a complete meal.

NUTRITIONAL VALUES PER SERVING (ASSUMING 4 SERVINGS):

Calories: 250 | Protein: 30g | Carbohydrates: 10g | Fat: 12g

Serving Portion: 1/4 of the skillet

Prep Time: 10 minutes

Cooking Time: 10 minutes

DIET RECIPE NOTE:

1. It prioritizes whole, unprocessed ingredients and is naturally low in added sugars and unhealthy fats. Shrimp and asparagus are both excellent sources of anti-inflammatory nutrients, including omega-3 fatty acids and antioxidants.

2. The use of olive oil further enhances the anti-inflammatory benefits of the meal. Additionally, the recipe is gluten-free and can be easily adapted to be dairy-free.

7. Caribbean Fish Stew

This Caribbean Fish Stew is a delicious and nutritious meal that can be a welcome addition to an RA-friendly diet. Bursting with fresh vegetables, aromatic spices, and hearty fish, this stew offers a delicious combination of tastes and textures. The use of fish, particularly those rich in omega-3 fatty acids, provides anti-inflammatory benefits, while the abundance of vegetables contributes essential vitamins, minerals, and antioxidants. It's a wholesome and satisfying meal that supports overall health and well-being.

INGREDIENTS:

- 1 tablespoon olive oil

- 1 medium onion, chopped

- 2 cloves garlic, minced

- 1 red bell pepper, chopped

- 1 green bell pepper, chopped

- 1 Scotch bonnet pepper, finely chopped (optional, remove seeds for less heat)

- 1 teaspoon ground cumin

- 1/2 teaspoon ground turmeric

- 1/4 teaspoon ground allspice

- 1 (14.5 ounces) can have diced tomatoes, undrained

- 1 cup vegetable broth or fish broth

- 1 pound firm white fish, cut into chunks (cod, halibut, or tilapia)

- 1/2 cup chopped fresh cilantro

- Salt and pepper to taste

- Lime wedges, for serving

PREPARATION METHODS:

1. Heat the olive oil in a large pot or Dutch oven over medium heat. Add the onion and cook until softened about 5 minutes.

2. Add the garlic, bell peppers, and Scotch bonnet pepper (if using) and cook for another 2-3 minutes, until the aroma comes out.

3. Stir in the cumin, turmeric, and allspice. Cook for 1 minute more, until the spices are aromatic.

4. Add the diced tomatoes, and vegetable broth, and bring to a cook.

5. Gently add the fish chunks to the pot and cook for 5-7 minutes, or until the fish is

cooked through and flakes easily with a fork.

PREP TIPS:

1. If you like a milder stew, omit the Scotch bonnet pepper or remove the seeds before chopping.

2. You can substitute the firm white fish with any other type of fish that you enjoy, such as salmon or mahi-mahi.

3. To make this recipe vegan, omit the fish and use vegetable broth instead of fish

6. Stir in the chopped cilantro and season with salt and pepper to taste.

7. Serve hot with lime wedges on the side.

broth. You can add more vegetables or plant-based protein sources like chickpeas or lentils.

4. Feel free to adjust the spices to your liking.

5. Serve with brown rice or quinoa for a complete meal.

NUTRITIONAL VALUES PER SERVING (ASSUMING 4 SERVINGS):

Calories: 300-350 (depending on the type of fish used) | Protein: 25-30g | Carbohydrates: 20-25g | Fat: 15-20g | Fiber: 5-7g

Serving Portion: 1 1/2 cups

Prep Time: 15 minutes

Cooking Time: 20-25 minutes

DIET RECIPE NOTE:

1. It prioritizes whole, unprocessed ingredients and is low in added sugars and unhealthy fats.
2. The fish provides a good source of omega-3 fatty acids, which have anti-inflammatory properties.
3. The vegetables offer essential vitamins, minerals, and antioxidants.

8. Spiced Trout and Vegetable Packets

T his recipe offers a simple yet spicy way to enjoy the benefits of fish and vegetables in one convenient package. The trout, a rich source of omega-3 fatty acids, provides anti-inflammatory benefits, while the colorful vegetables add vitamins, minerals, and antioxidants to the mix. The spices help the taste without relying on excessive salt or unhealthy fats, making this a nutritious and delicious option for people with rheumatoid arthritis.

INGREDIENTS:

- 4 trout fillets (about 6 ounces each)
- 1 tablespoon olive oil
- 1 teaspoon ground cumin
- 1/2 teaspoon ground coriander
- 1/4 teaspoon turmeric powder
- 1/4 teaspoon garlic powder
- 1/4 teaspoon salt
- 1/4 teaspoon black pepper
- 1 zucchini, thinly sliced
- 1 yellow squash, thinly sliced
- 1 red bell pepper, thinly sliced
- 1/2 cup cherry tomatoes, halved
- 1/4 cup chopped fresh parsley
- Lemon wedges, for serving

PREPARATION METHOD:

1. Heat oven to 400°F (200°C).

2. Cut four large sheets of aluminum foil.

3. In a small bowl, mix the olive oil, cumin, coriander, turmeric, garlic powder, salt, and pepper.

4. Place one trout fillet in the center of each foil sheet.

5. Sprinkle the spice mixture over each fillet.

6. Top with zucchini, yellow squash, bell pepper, and cherry tomatoes. Divide the parsley equally among the packets.

7. Bring the sides of the foil together and fold to create a sealed packet, leaving some space for steam to circulate.

8. Place the packets on a baking sheet and bake for 15-20 minutes, or until the fish is cooked through and flakes easily with a fork.

9. Carefully open the packets and serve immediately with lemon wedges.

PREP TIPS:

1. You can substitute trout with other types of fish like salmon or cod.

2. Feel free to try different vegetables, such as broccoli florets, asparagus spears, or green beans.

3. Add a squeeze of lemon juice to the packets before sealing for more taste.

4. If you prefer a spicier meal, add a pinch of cayenne pepper or red pepper flakes to the spice mixture.

NUTRITIONAL VALUES PER SERVING (1 PACKET):

Calories: 350-400 | Protein: 30-35g | Carbohydrates: 20-25g | Fat: 15-20g

Serving Portion: 1 packet

Prep Time: 15 minutes

Cooking Time: 15-20 minutes

DIET RECIPE NOTE:

1. It emphasizes whole, unprocessed ingredients and utilizes healthy cooking methods. The trout is a good source of omega-3 fatty acids, which have anti-inflammatory properties.
2. The vegetables offer essential vitamins, minerals, and antioxidants. The spices enhance the flavor without the need for excessive salt or unhealthy fats.
3. It's a balanced meal with protein, healthy fats, and complex carbohydrates.

9. Almond-Crusted Halibut

Almond-Crusted Halibut is a delicious meal that marries the delicate taste of halibut with a crunchy, nutty crust. It's a good option for people with rheumatoid arthritis as it features anti-inflammatory ingredients and a cooking method that preserves the nutrients and healthy fats in the fish. The almonds provide a good source of protein, fiber, and healthy fats, while halibut is rich in omega-3 fatty acids, known for their anti-inflammatory properties.

INGREDIENTS:

- 4 halibut fillets (about 6 ounces each)

- 1/2 cup almond flour

- 1/4 cup chopped fresh parsley

- 1/4 teaspoon garlic powder

- 1/4 teaspoon onion powder

- 1/4 teaspoon salt

- 1/8 teaspoon black pepper

- 2 tablespoons olive oil

- Lemon wedges, for serving

PREPARATION METHODS:

1. Heat oven to 400°F (200°C). Line a baking sheet with parchment paper.

2. In a shallow bowl, combine the almond flour, parsley, garlic powder, onion powder, salt, and pepper.

3. Pat the halibut fillets dry with paper towels.

4. Sprinkle the halibut fillets with olive oil and season both sides with salt and pepper.

5. Dredge each fillet in the almond flour mixture, pressing to coat evenly.

6. Place the fillets on the prepared baking sheet.

7. Bake for 12-15 minutes, or until the fish is cooked through and flakes easily with a fork.

8. Serve immediately with lemon wedges.

PREP TIPS:

1. To ensure a crispy crust, make sure the halibut fillets are dry before coating them in the almond flour mixture.

2. You can substitute almond flour with other nut flour like hazelnut or walnut flour.

3. Feel free to add other herbs and spices to the almond flour mixture, such as dried thyme or paprika.

4. For a richer taste, sprinkle the finished halibut with a small amount of melted ghee or olive oil.

5. Serve with a side of steamed vegetables or a fresh salad for a complete meal.

NUTRITIONAL VALUES PER SERVING:

Calories: 350 | Protein: 35g | Carbohydrates: 10g | Fat: 20g | Fiber: 3g

Serving Portion: 1 halibut fillet

Prep Time: 10 minutes

Cooking Time: 12-15 minutes

DIET RECIPE NOTE:

1. This Almond-Crusted Halibut recipe is well-suited for an RA-friendly diet. It prioritizes whole, unprocessed ingredients and is naturally low in added sugars and sodium.
2. The use of almond flour provides a good source of protein, fiber, and healthy fats. Halibut is a lean protein source rich in omega-3 fatty acids, which have anti-inflammatory properties.
3. Baking the fish helps to preserve its nutrients and avoids the use of excessive oil.

10. Spiced Grilled Chicken with Cauliflower "Rice" Tabbouleh

This delicious and nutritious meal is a fantastic addition to an RA-friendly diet. It combines the lean protein of grilled chicken with the wholesome goodness of cauliflower "rice" tabbouleh, a light and refreshing salad rich in anti-inflammatory ingredients. The spices used in the chicken marinade not only help the taste but may also offer additional anti-inflammatory benefits.

INGREDIENTS:

FOR THE CHICKEN:

- 1 pound boneless, skinless chicken breasts

- 2 1/2 teaspoons ground cumin, divided

- 1 1/2 teaspoons dried marjoram

- 3/4 teaspoon salt, divided

- 1/4 teaspoon ground allspice

- 1/4 teaspoon cayenne pepper

- 2 tablespoons extra-virgin olive oil

FOR THE TABBOULEH:

- 1/4 cup lemon juice

- 3 tablespoons extra-virgin olive oil

- 1/2 teaspoon ground cumin

- 1/4 teaspoon salt

- 2 cups fresh riced cauliflower

- 2 cups flat-leaf parsley leaves, chopped

- 1 cup diced cucumber

- 1 cup halved cherry tomatoes

- ¼ cup sliced scallions

PREPARATION METHODS:

1. Heat the grill to medium-high heat.

2. In a small bowl, combine 2 tablespoons olive oil, 2 teaspoons cumin, marjoram, 1/2 teaspoon salt, allspice, and cayenne pepper.

3. Brush the chicken breasts with the spice mixture.

4. Grill the chicken, turning occasionally, until an instant-read thermometer inserted into the thickest part registers 165°F (74°C), about 10-12 minutes.

5. Remove the chicken from the grill and let it rest for 5 minutes before slicing.

6. While the chicken is grilling, mix the lemon juice, 3 tablespoons olive oil, 1/2 teaspoon cumin, and 1/4 teaspoon salt in a large bowl.

7. Add the rice cauliflower, parsley, cucumber, tomatoes, and scallions to the bowl. Toss to coat well.

8. Thinly slice the rested chicken.

9. Serve the chicken slices over the cauliflower tabbouleh.

PREP TIPS:

1. To make riced cauliflower, pulse cauliflower florets in a food processor until they resemble rice grains. Alternatively, you can grate the cauliflower using a box grater.

2. If you don't have a grill, you can cook the chicken in a pan over medium-high heat.

3. Feel free to adjust the spices in the chicken marinade to your liking.

4. Add other vegetables to the tabbouleh, such as chopped bell peppers or diced zucchini.

NUTRITIONAL VALUES PER SERVING (ASSUMING 4 SERVINGS):

Calories: 350 | Protein: 30g | Carbohydrates: 25g | Fat: 18g | Fiber: 5g

Serving Portion: 1 chicken breast with 1 cup of tabbouleh

Prep Time: 15 minutes

Cooking Time: 10-12 minutes

DIET RECIPE NOTE:

1. This recipe aligns well with an RA-friendly diet. It emphasizes lean protein (chicken), vegetables, and healthy fats (olive oil).

2. Cauliflower "rice" provides a low-carb, nutrient-rich option to local grains. The spices used may offer additional anti-inflammatory benefits.

3. The recipe is naturally free of added sugars and can be easily adjusted to reduce sodium by using less salt.

11. Halibut with Gingered Slaw and Avocado

This delicious and nutritious meal is a delightful addition to an RA-friendly diet. The star of the show, halibut, is lean fish rich in omega-3 fatty acids, renowned for their anti-inflammatory properties. It is complemented by a refreshing gingered slaw, rich in crunchy vegetables and a zesty dressing, further boosting the anti-inflammatory potential of the meal. The creamy avocado adds healthy fats and a satisfying texture, making this dish a nourishing and delicious choice for those managing rheumatoid arthritis.

INGREDIENTS:

FOR THE HALIBUT:

- 4 halibut fillets (about 6 oz each)
- 1 tablespoon olive oil
- 1/2 teaspoon grated fresh ginger
- 1/4 teaspoon salt
- 1/4 teaspoon black pepper

FOR THE GINGERED SLAW:

- 2 cups shredded green cabbage
- 1 cup shredded red cabbage
- 1/2 cup shredded carrots

- 1/4 cup chopped fresh cilantro
- 2 tablespoons rice vinegar
- 1 tablespoon olive oil
- 1 tablespoon grated fresh ginger
- 1 teaspoon honey (or maple syrup)
- 1/2 teaspoon salt
- 1/4 teaspoon black pepper

FOR SERVING:

- 1 ripe avocado, sliced

PREPARATION METHODS:

1. In a large bowl, combine the shredded cabbage, carrots, and cilantro. In a separate small bowl, mix the rice vinegar, olive oil, ginger, honey (or maple syrup), salt, and pepper. Pour the dressing over the slaw and toss to coat evenly.

2. Pat the halibut fillets dry with paper towels. In a small bowl, combine the olive oil, ginger, salt, and pepper. Brush the halibut fillets with the olive oil mixture.

3. Heat a large pan over medium-high heat. Add the halibut fillets and cook for about 4-5 minutes per side, or until cooked through and flakes easily with a fork.

4. Divide the gingered slaw among four plates. Top with the cooked halibut fillets and sliced avocado. Enjoy immediately!

PREP TIPS:

1. You can prepare the gingered slaw ahead of time and store it in the refrigerator for up to 3 days.

2. Feel free to substitute halibut with other types of fish like salmon or cod.

3. If you don't have rice vinegar, you can use apple cider vinegar or white wine vinegar.

4. To make this recipe vegan, omit the honey or maple syrup from the slaw dressing or substitute with agave nectar.

NUTRITIONAL VALUES PER SERVING:

Calories: 400-450 | Protein: 30-35g | Carbohydrates: 25-30g | Fat: 20-25g | Fiber: 5-7g

Serving Portion: 1 halibut fillet with slaw and avocado

Prep Time: 20 minutes

Cooking Time: 8-10 minutes

DIET RECIPE NOTE:

1. It focuses on whole, unprocessed ingredients and is low in added sugars and unhealthy fats. The halibut provides a good source of omega-3 fatty acids, which have anti-inflammatory properties.
2. The gingered slaw offers a variety of vitamins, minerals, and antioxidants that further support a healthy immune system. The avocado adds healthy fats and fiber, contributing to a feeling of fullness and satisfaction.

12. Herb and Walnut–Crusted Pork Chops

This recipe offers a great twist on classic pork chops, creating a delicious and nutritious meal suitable for individuals managing rheumatoid arthritis. The herb and walnut crust add a satisfying crunch and a burst of anti-inflammatory compounds. While pork is generally recommended in moderation for an RA diet, choosing lean cuts and pairing them with plenty of vegetables can make this a healthy and enjoyable meal option.

INGREDIENTS:

- 4 boneless, center-cut pork chops (about 1 inch thick)

- 1/2 cup walnuts, finely chopped

- 1/4 cup fresh parsley, chopped

- 1/4 cup fresh rosemary, chopped

- 1 tablespoon olive oil

- 1/2 teaspoon salt

- 1/4 teaspoon black pepper

PREPARATION METHODS:

1. Heat oven to 400°F (200°C). Line a baking sheet with parchment paper.

2. In a shallow bowl, combine the chopped walnuts, parsley, rosemary, olive oil, salt, and pepper. Mix well.

3. Press each pork chop into the walnut mixture, coating both sides evenly.

4. Place the coated pork chops on the prepared baking sheet.

5. Bake for 15-20 minutes, or until the internal temperature reaches 145°F (63°C).

6. Let the pork chops rest for a few minutes before serving.

PREP TIPS:

1. To ensure even cooking, choose pork chops that are similar in thickness.

2. You can substitute walnuts with other nuts like almonds or pecans.

3. Feel free to try different herbs, such as thyme or oregano.

4. Serve the pork chops with a side of roasted vegetables or a fresh salad for a complete meal.

NUTRITIONAL VALUES PER SERVING (1 PORK CHOP):

Calories: 350-400 (depending on the size of the pork chop) | Protein: 30-35g | Carbohydrates: 10-15g | Fat: 20-25g

Serving Portion: 1 pork chop

Prep Time: 10 minutes

Cooking Time: 15-20 minutes

DIET RECIPE NOTE:

1. Pork, especially red meat, should be consumed in moderation due to its potential to increase inflammation. Enjoy this meal occasionally as part of a balanced meal.

2. Choose center-cut pork chops, which are leaner than other cuts. Trim any visible fat before cooking.

3. Pair the pork chops with plenty of vegetables, such as roasted Brussels sprouts or a side salad, to increase the nutrient density and fiber content of the meal.

4. The walnuts and olive oil provide healthy fats, which are important for overall health and can help reduce inflammation.

5. The fresh herbs add flavor and potential anti-inflammatory benefits.

13. Italian Sausage and Kale Soup

This tasty and nutritious Italian Sausage and Kale Soup is a comforting and nutritious meal that can be easily adapted to fit an RA-friendly diet. It combines lean protein from Italian sausage with the anti-inflammatory benefits of kale and other vegetables. The warmth and spices of this soup make it a satisfying option, particularly during colder months, while the nutrient-rich ingredients support overall health and well-being.

INGREDIENTS:

- 1 pound Italian sausage (choose a lean variety, preferably chicken or turkey)

- 1 tablespoon olive oil

- 1 medium onion, chopped

- 2 cloves garlic, minced

- 4 cups low-sodium chicken broth or vegetable broth

- 1 (14.5 ounces) can of diced tomatoes, undrained

- 1 bunch of kale, stemmed and chopped

- 1/2 teaspoon dried oregano

- 1/4 teaspoon red pepper flakes (optional)

- Salt and pepper to taste

PREPARATION METHODS:

1. In a large pot, brown the sausage over medium heat, breaking it up with a spoon as it cooks.

2. Remove the sausage from the pot and set aside.

3. Add the olive oil to the pot and sauté the onion until softened about 5 minutes. Add the garlic and cook for an additional minute, until the aroma comes out.

4. Return the sausage to the pot, then add the broth, diced tomatoes, kale, oregano, and red pepper flakes (if using). Season with salt and pepper to taste.

5. Bring the soup to a boil, then reduce heat to low and cook for 15-20 minutes, or until the kale is soft.

PREP TIPS:

1. To make this recipe even healthier, use ground turkey or chicken instead of sausage.

2. If you like a vegetarian option, omit the sausage and add additional vegetables or beans.

3. Feel free to substitute kale with other leafy greens like spinach or Swiss chard.

4. For a creamier soup, add a splash of heavy cream or coconut milk at the end.

5. Serve with a slice of whole-grain bread for a complete meal.

NUTRITIONAL VALUES PER SERVING (ASSUMING 4 SERVINGS):

Calories: 300-350 (depending on the sausage and broth used) | Protein: 20-25g | Carbohydrates: 20-25g | Fat: 15-20g | Fiber: 5-7g

Serving Portion: 1 1/2 - 2 cups

Prep Time: 15 minutes

Cooking Time: 20-25 minutes

DIET RECIPE NOTE:

1. The key is to choose a lean variety of Italian sausage, preferably chicken or turkey, to limit saturated fat intake. Option for low-sodium broth to reduce sodium content.

2. Kale is a great source of anti-inflammatory nutrients, and other vegetables add vitamins and minerals.

3. Be mindful of the oil used and avoid deep-frying the sausage. This recipe is naturally gluten-free. If nightshades are a concern, omit the tomatoes and red pepper flakes.

14. Lamb Burgers with Papaya Salsa

These Lamb Burgers with Papaya Salsa offer a good twist on a classic favorite, making it a suitable and delicious option for individuals managing rheumatoid arthritis. Lean ground lamb provides a good source of protein and essential nutrients, while papaya salsa adds a burst of tropical sweetness and anti-inflammatory benefits. The combination of lean protein, fruits, and vegetables makes this meal a well-rounded and nourishing meal.

INGREDIENTS:

FOR THE LAMB BURGERS:

- 1 pound ground lamb (choose a lean ground lamb or drain excess fat after cooking)

- 1/4 cup finely chopped onion

- 1/4 cup finely chopped fresh parsley

- 1 tablespoon Worcestershire sauce (check for gluten-free if needed)

- 1 teaspoon ground cumin

- 1/2 teaspoon salt

- 1/4 teaspoon black pepper

FOR THE PAPAYA SALSA:

- 1 ripe papaya, peeled, seeded, and diced

- 1/2 cup diced red bell pepper

- 1/4 cup diced red onion

- 1/4 cup chopped fresh cilantro

- 1 tablespoon lime juice

- Salt and pepper to taste

- **Optional:** Whole-grain buns or lettuce wraps

PREPARATION METHODS:

1. In a large bowl, combine the ground lamb, onion, parsley, Worcestershire sauce, cumin, salt, and pepper. Gently mix until just combined, being careful not to overwork the meat. Shape the mixture into 4 patties, about 1 inch thick.

2. In a medium bowl, combine the diced papaya, red bell pepper, red onion, cilantro, and lime juice. Season with salt and pepper to taste.

3. Heat a grill or pan over medium heat. Cook the lamb burgers for about 5-7

minutes per side, or until they reach an internal temperature of 160°F.

4. If using buns, lightly toast them. Place a lamb burger on each bun or lettuce wrap. Top with a generous scoop of papaya salsa. Serve immediately.

PREP TIPS:

1. You can make the papaya salsa ahead of time and store it in the refrigerator until ready to use.

2. If you don't have a grill, you can cook the burgers in a pan on the stovetop.

3. To add more taste, try marinating the lamb patties in a mixture of olive oil, lemon juice, and herbs for 30 minutes to an hour before grilling.

4. For a spicier salsa, add a pinch of chopped jalapeño or red pepper flakes.

NUTRITIONAL VALUES PER SERVING (1 BURGER WITH SALSA, WITHOUT BUN):

Calories: 350-400 (depending on the fat content of the lamb) | Protein: 25-30g | Carbohydrates: 20-25g | Fat: 20-25g | Fiber: 3-4g

Serving Portion: 1 burger with salsa

Prep Time: 20 minutes

Cooking Time: 10-14 minutes

DIET RECIPE NOTE:

1. This recipe can be suitable for an RA-friendly diet with some modifications. Option for lean ground lamb or drain excess fat after cooking to limit saturated fat intake.

2. The papaya salsa adds a boost of vitamins, minerals, and antioxidants. If using buns, choose whole-grain options for added fiber and nutrients.

15. Taco Bowl with Cauliflower Rice and Avocado

This delicious and nutritious Taco Bowl with Cauliflower Rice and Avocado is a nice addition to an RA-friendly diet. It's a wholesome, selected meal that provides a satisfying balance of protein, fiber, and healthy fats, all while being low in inflammatory triggers. The cauliflower rice offers a lighter option to local rice, while the avocado adds creaminess and essential nutrients. It's a delicious and nutritious option for lunch or dinner.

INGREDIENTS:

FOR THE CAULIFLOWER RICE:

- 1 head of cauliflower, riced (about 4 cups)
- 1 tablespoon olive oil
- 1/2 teaspoon ground cumin
- 1/4 teaspoon chili powder
- Salt and pepper to taste

FOR THE TACO FILLING:

- 1 pound ground turkey or chicken (or plant-based alternative)
- 1 onion, chopped
- 1 bell pepper, chopped

- 1 (15 ounces) can of black beans, rinsed and drained
- 1 (10 ounces) can dice tomatoes and green chilies, undrained
- 1 tablespoon taco seasoning

TOPPINGS:

- 1 avocado, sliced or diced
- Shredded lettuce
- Chopped tomatoes
- Chopped cilantro
- Lime wedges

PREPARATION METHODS:

1. Heat the olive oil in a large pan over medium heat. Add the rice cauliflower, cumin, chili powder, salt, and pepper. Cook, stirring occasionally, until the cauliflower is soft-crisp, about 5-7 minutes.

2. In a separate pan, brown the ground turkey or chicken (or cook your plant-based option according to package instructions) over medium heat. Add the onion and bell pepper and cook until softened about 5 minutes.

3. Stir in the black beans, diced tomatoes green chilies, and taco seasoning. Bring to a simmer and cook for 5 minutes, or until heated through.

4. Divide the cauliflower rice among bowls. Top with the taco filling, avocado slices, shredded lettuce, chopped tomatoes, cilantro, and a squeeze of lime.

PREP TIPS:

1. You can buy pre-riced cauliflower or rice on your own using a food processor or grater.

2. To add more spice, use a hotter taco seasoning or add a pinch of cayenne pepper to the filling.

3. Make your bowls with your favorite toppings, such as salsa, shredded cheese (in moderation), or pickled onions.

4. Make a big batch of the filling and cauliflower rice ahead of time for quick and easy meals throughout the week.

NUTRITIONAL VALUES PER SERVING (ASSUMING 4 SERVINGS):

Calories: 400-450 (depending on toppings) | Protein: 30-35g | Carbohydrates: 35-40g | Fat: 20-25g | Fiber: 10-12g

Serving Portion: 1 bowl

Prep Time: 20 minutes

Cooking Time: 15-20 minutes

DIET RECIPE NOTE:

1. It emphasizes whole, unprocessed ingredients and is naturally low in added sugars and unhealthy fats.

2. The cauliflower rice provides a good source of fiber and vitamins, while the lean protein and avocado offer essential nutrients.

3. This recipe is also gluten-free and can be easily adapted to be vegan by using plant-based protein options.

Self-Reflection Questions:

1. What are my current dinner habits, and how do they align with an anti-inflammatory approach?

_____

_____

_____

_____

_____

_____

2. Which RA-friendly dinner recipes appeal to me the most, and why?

_____

_____

_____

_____

_____

3. What challenges do I face when preparing dinner, especially on days when my RA symptoms are flaring up?

_____

_____

_____

_____

_____

4. How can I make dinnertime a more mindful and enjoyable experience, even when I'm feeling fatigued or in pain?

_____

_____

_____

_____

_____

5. What are my goals for incorporating more anti-inflammatory dinners into my routine, and how will I track my progress and celebrate my successes?

_____

_____

_____

_____

_____

_____

_____

_____

_____

_____

_____

_____

_____

_____

_____

CHAPTER 6:
RA-FRIENDLY DESSERT & SNACK DIET

1. Almond-Quinoa Crisps

Almond-Quinoa Crisps offers a delicious and nutritious snack option that perfectly complements an RA-friendly diet. These crispy treats are rich in protein, fiber, and healthy fats, making them a satisfying and energizing snack to curb cravings and support overall well-being. The combination of almonds and quinoa provides a rich source of anti-inflammatory nutrients, making them an excellent choice for individuals managing rheumatoid arthritis.

INGREDIENTS:

- 1 cup cooked quinoa, cooled

- 1/2 cup almond flour

- 1/4 cup chopped almonds

- 1/4 cup pumpkin seeds

- 1/4 cup sunflower seeds

- 2 tablespoons olive oil

- 1 tablespoon maple syrup (or other natural sweetener)

- 1/2 teaspoon ground cinnamon

- 1/4 teaspoon salt

PREPARATION METHODS:

1. Heat oven to 350°F (175°C). Line a baking sheet with parchment paper.

2. In a large bowl, combine the cooked quinoa, almond flour, chopped almonds, pumpkin seeds, sunflower seeds, olive oil, maple syrup, cinnamon, and salt. Mix well until all ingredients are evenly incorporated.

3. Spread the mixture onto the prepared baking sheet in a thin, even layer. You can

use the back of a spoon or your hands to press it down.

4. Bake for 20-25 minutes, or until the crisps are golden brown and crispy.

5. Let cool completely on the baking sheet before breaking into pieces.

PREP TIPS:

1. You can cook the quinoa ahead of time to save on preparation time.

2. Feel free to substitute the almonds, pumpkin seeds, and sunflower seeds with other nuts or seeds of your choice.

3. For a sweeter crisp, add a more tablespoon of maple syrup or sprinkle with honey after baking.

4. Store the crisps in an airtight container at room temperature for up to 3 days.

NUTRITIONAL VALUES PER SERVING (APPROXIMATELY 12 CRISPS):

Calories: 150-170 | Protein: 5-7g | Carbohydrates: 18-20g | Fat: 8-10g | Fiber: 3-4g

Serving Portion: 12 crisps

Prep Time: 15 minutes

Cooking Time: 20-25 minutes

DIET RECIPE NOTE:

1. They are made with whole, unprocessed ingredients and are naturally low in added sugars and unhealthy fats.

2. Quinoa and almonds provide protein, fiber, and healthy fats, while the seeds add more nutrients and crunch.

3. This recipe is also gluten-free and can be easily adapted to be vegan by using a plant-based sweetener like agave nectar or maple syrup.

2. Blackberry-Lemon Granita

Blackberry-Lemon Granita is a refreshing and healthy frozen dessert great for individuals with rheumatoid arthritis. It's a simple, naturally sweet treat bursting with antioxidants from blackberries and a touch of citrusy tang from lemon. This recipe is free from processed ingredients, added sugars, and unhealthy fats, making it a guilt-free indulgence that supports an anti-inflammatory diet.

INGREDIENTS:

- 3 cups fresh or frozen blackberries

- 1/2 cup water

- 1/4 cup freshly squeezed lemon juice

- 1-2 tablespoons honey or maple syrup (adjust to taste)

PREPARATION METHODS:

1. Combine the blackberries, water, lemon juice, and sweetener in a blender or food processor. Blend until smooth.

2. If you prefer a smoother texture, strain the mixture through a fine-mesh sieve to remove any seeds.

3. Pour the mixture into a shallow bowl or baking pan. Cover with plastic wrap and freeze for 1-2 hours, or until partially frozen.

4. Using a fork, scrape the granita to break up the ice crystals. Return to the freezer.

5. Continue scraping the granita every 30-60 minutes until it is completely frozen and has a light, flaky texture. This may take 3-4 hours.

6. Scoop the granita into bowls or glasses and enjoy immediately.

PREP TIPS:

1. For a more intense taste, use frozen blackberries.

2. If you don't have fresh lemon juice, you can use bottled lemon juice, but make sure it's 100% pure juice with no added sugars.

3. If you want to make this recipe vegan, use maple syrup or agave nectar instead of honey.

4. To add a touch of importance, garnish with fresh mint leaves or a sprinkle of lemon zest.

NUTRITIONAL VALUES PER SERVING (ASSUMING 4 SERVINGS):

Calories: 100-120 (depending on the sweetener used) | Protein: 1g | Carbohydrates: 25-30g | Fat: 0-1g | Fiber: 3-4g

Serving Portion: 1/2 cup

Prep Time: 10 minutes (freezing time 3-4 hours)

DIET RECIPE NOTE:

1. It is made with whole, unprocessed ingredients and is naturally sweetened with honey or maple syrup.
2. Blackberries are rich in antioxidants, which can help combat inflammation. Lemon juice adds vitamin C, another powerful antioxidant.
3. This recipe is also gluten-free, and dairy-free, and can be easily adapted to be vegan.

_____

_____

_____

_____

_____

_____

_____

_____

3. Tangy Lemon Mousse

This light and refreshing Tangy Lemon Mousse offers a delicious dessert option that aligns well with an RA-friendly diet. It boasts a vibrant citrus taste and a smooth, airy texture, making it a guilt-free option. The recipe focuses on natural ingredients, avoiding processed elements and refined sugars, which can trigger inflammation. Lemons, rich in vitamin C and antioxidants, add a tangy twist while potentially offering anti-inflammatory benefits.

INGREDIENTS:

- 1 cup heavy cream (or a dairy-free option like coconut cream)

- 1/4 cup freshly squeezed lemon juice

- 1/4 cup honey or maple syrup (adjust to taste)

- Zest of 1 lemon

- Pinch of salt

PREPARATION METHODS:

1. In a chilled bowl, beat the heavy cream (or dairy-free option) with an electric mixer until stiff peaks form.

2. In a separate bowl, mix the lemon juice, honey (or maple syrup), lemon zest, and salt.

3. Gently fold the lemon mixture into the whipped cream until just combined. Be careful not to overmix, or the mousse will deflate.

4. Divide the mousse into serving meals and refrigerate for at least 2 hours, or until set.

5. Garnish with additional lemon zest or fresh berries, if desired.

PREP TIPS:

1. Make sure the bowl and beaters are chilled before whipping the cream. This will help it whip up faster and hold its shape better.

2. Use fresh lemons for the best flavor and aroma.

3. Taste the lemon mixture before folding it into the whipped cream and adjust the sweetness as needed.

4. For a vegan option, use a plant-based whipped cream alternative and agar agar powder as a thickener.

5. If you don't have honey or maple syrup, you can use another natural sweetener like agave nectar or coconut sugar.

NUTRITIONAL VALUES PER SERVING (ASSUMING 4 SERVINGS):

Calories: 250-300 (depending on the type of cream and sweetener used) | Protein: 2-3g | Carbohydrates: 25-30g | Fat: 20-25g

Serving Portion: 1/2 cup

Prep Time: 15 minutes (refrigeration time required)

DIET RECIPE NOTE:

1. It utilizes natural ingredients and avoids processed elements and refined sugars. The use of lemon and its zest potentially provides anti-inflammatory benefits.
2. However, individuals with sensitivities to dairy or high-fat foods might want to consider using a dairy-free cream option or adjusting the portion size accordingly.

---

4. Blueberry-Fig Open-Face Pie

This delicious Blueberry-Fig Open-Face Pie offers a burst of taste and a visual treat, making it a great dessert or snack option for individuals with rheumatoid arthritis. Bursting with antioxidants from blueberries and figs, this pie utilizes a healthier crust and natural sweeteners, ensuring it aligns well with an anti-inflammatory diet.

INGREDIENTS:

FOR THE CRUST:

- 1 cup almond flour
- 1/4 cup coconut flour
- 1/4 cup rolled oats
- 1/4 teaspoon salt
- 3 tablespoons coconut oil, melted
- 2 tablespoons maple syrup

FOR THE FILLING:

- 2 cups fresh or frozen blueberries
- 1 cup fresh or dried figs, chopped
- 1 tablespoon lemon juice
- 1 tablespoon cornstarch or tapioca starch
- 1/4 cup maple syrup (or adjust to taste)
- 1/4 teaspoon ground cinnamon

PREPARATION METHODS:

1. Heat your oven to 350°F (175°C).

2. In a medium bowl, combine the almond flour, coconut flour, oats, and salt.

3. Add the melted coconut oil and maple syrup and mix until a dough forms.

4. Press the dough into the bottom of a 9-inch pie bowl or tart pan.

5. Bake for 10-12 minutes, or until lightly golden.

6. In a large bowl, combine the blueberries, figs, lemon juice, cornstarch (or tapioca starch), maple syrup, and cinnamon. Toss gently to coat.

7. Pour the filling into the pre-baked crust.

8. Bake for 20-25 minutes, or until the filling is bubbly and the crust is golden brown.

9. Let cool slightly before serving.

PREP TIPS:

1. If using dried figs, soak them in warm water for 15-20 minutes before chopping to plump them up.

2. You can substitute the almond flour with another nut flour, such as hazelnut or walnut flour.

3. If you like a sweeter pie, increase the amount of maple syrup in the filling.

4. Serve the pie warm with a dollop of coconut yogurt or a scoop of vanilla ice cream (optional).

NUTRITIONAL VALUES PER SERVING (ASSUMING 8 SERVINGS):

Calories: 250-300 (depending on the sweetness and toppings) | Protein: 5-7g | Carbohydrates: 30-35g | Fat: 15-18g | Fiber: 5-7g

Serving Portion: 1 slice

Prep Time: 20 minutes

Cooking Time: 30-35 minutes

DIET RECIPE NOTE:

1. It prioritizes whole, unprocessed ingredients and avoids refined sugars and flours. The almond and coconut flour crust is a healthier option to local pastry, and the natural sweetness from maple syrup is a better choice than refined sugar.

2. The blueberries and figs provide a rich source of antioxidants, which can help combat inflammation.

_____

_____

_____

_____

_____

_____

5. Berry-Rhubarb Cobbler

A delicious combination of the sweet and tart taste, this Berry-Rhubarb Cobbler offers a comforting and nutritious dessert option for those following an RA-friendly diet. Bursting with antioxidants from berries and rhubarb, this cobbler provides a satisfying treat without the inflammatory triggers found in many local desserts. The simple biscuit topping, made with wholesome ingredients, adds a touch of warmth and texture.

INGREDIENTS:

FOR THE FILLING:

- 4 cups mixed berries (fresh or frozen, such as strawberries, blueberries, raspberries)

- 2 cups chopped rhubarb

- 1/2 cup maple syrup or coconut sugar

- 1/4 cup cornstarch

- 1 tablespoon lemon juice

- 1/2 teaspoon ground cinnamon

FOR THE BISCUIT TOPPING:

- 1 cup whole wheat flour (or gluten-free blend)

- 1/2 cup almond flour

- 1/4 cup maple syrup or coconut sugar

- 2 teaspoons baking powder

- 1/2 teaspoon baking soda

- 1/4 teaspoon salt

- 1/4 cup unsweetened applesauce

- 1/4 cup milk (dairy or plant-based)

- 1 tablespoon melted coconut oil

PREPARATION METHODS:

1. Heat oven to 375°F (190°C).

2. In a large bowl, combine the berries, rhubarb, maple syrup (or coconut sugar), cornstarch, lemon juice, and cinnamon. Toss to coat evenly.

3. In a separate bowl, mix the whole wheat flour, almond flour, maple syrup (or coconut sugar), baking powder, baking soda, and salt.

4. In a small bowl, mix the applesauce, milk, and melted coconut oil.

5. Add the wet ingredients to the dry ingredients and stir until just combined.

Be careful not to overmix. The dough should be slightly sticky.

6. Pour the berry-rhubarb filling into a 9x13-inch baking dish. Drop a spoonful of the biscuit topping over the fruit mixture.

7. Bake for 30-35 minutes, or until the topping is golden brown and the filling is bubbling.

8. Let the cobbler cool slightly before serving warm with a scoop of vanilla yogurt or ice cream (optional).

PREP TIPS:

1. If using frozen berries, thaw them slightly before using.

2. You can adjust the sweetness of the filling and topping by adding more or less maple syrup or coconut sugar.

3. For a crispier topping, sprinkle a tablespoon of turbinado sugar over the biscuits before baking.

4. Feel free to try different types of berries and other fruits.

5. This cobbler is best served warm but can also be enjoyed at room temperature.

NUTRITIONAL VALUES PER SERVING (ASSUMING 12 SERVINGS):

Calories: 250 | Protein: 5g | Carbohydrates: 45g | Fat: 8g | Fiber: 5g

Serving Portion: 1/12 of the cobbler

Prep Time: 20 minutes   **Cooking Time:** 30-35 minutes

DIET RECIPE NOTE:

- If dairy is a concern, use a plant-based milk and yogurt alternative.

- Adjust the amount of sweetener to your liking, keeping in mind that added sugars should be limited in an RA diet.

- Some individuals with RA may be sensitive to nightshades. If this is the case, consider omitting the tomatoes from the recipe or replacing them with another fruit.

6. Maple Carrot Cake

A delicious and comforting treat, this Maple Carrot Cake offers a healthier twist on a classic dessert, making it suitable for those with rheumatoid arthritis. It incorporates anti-inflammatory ingredients like carrots, whole grains, and natural sweeteners while avoiding refined sugars and unhealthy fats. The warm spices and natural sweetness of maple syrup create a comforting and satisfying flavor profile that's perfect for any occasion.

INGREDIENTS:

- 2 cups finely grated carrots

- 1 1/2 cups whole wheat flour or gluten-free 1:1 baking flour

- 1 teaspoon baking powder

- 1/2 teaspoon baking soda

- 1/2 teaspoon salt

- 1 teaspoon ground cinnamon

- 1/2 teaspoon ground ginger

- 1/4 teaspoon ground nutmeg

- 3 large eggs

- 1/2 cup unsweetened applesauce

- 1/2 cup pure maple syrup

- 1/4 cup melted coconut oil

- 1 teaspoon vanilla extract

- 1/2 cup chopped walnuts or pecans (optional)

FOR THE CREAM CHEESE FROSTING (OPTIONAL):

- 4 ounces cream cheese, softened

- 2 tablespoons unsalted butter, softened

- 1/4 cup pure maple syrup

- 1/2 teaspoon vanilla extract

PREPARATION METHODS:

1. Heat oven to 350°F (175°C). Grease and flour a 9x13-inch baking pan.

2. In a large bowl, mix the flour, baking powder, baking soda, salt, cinnamon, ginger, and nutmeg.

3. In a separate bowl, mix the eggs, applesauce, maple syrup, melted coconut oil, and vanilla extract.

4. Gradually add the wet ingredients to the dry ingredients, mixing until just combined.

5. Fold in the grated carrots and nuts (if using).

6. Pour the batter into the prepared pan and bake for 30-35 minutes, or until a toothpick inserted into the center comes out clean.

7. Let the cake cool completely before frosting.

TO MAKE THE FROSTING (Optional):

1. In a medium bowl, beat together the cream cheese and butter until smooth and creamy.

2. Gradually add the maple syrup and vanilla extract, beating until well combined.

3. Frost the cooled cake as desired.

PREP TIPS:

1. For a richer taste, toast the nuts before adding them to the batter.

2. You can substitute applesauce with mashed banana or Greek yogurt.

3. If you like a denser cake, add an extra 1/4 cup of flour.

4. To make this recipe vegan, use flax eggs (1 tablespoon ground flaxseed + 3 tablespoons water) as an egg substitute and vegan cream cheese and butter alternatives for the frosting.

NUTRITIONAL VALUES PER SERVING (ASSUMING 12 SERVINGS):

Calories: 250-300 (depending on frosting) | Protein: 5-7g | Carbohydrates: 35-40g | Fat: 12-15g | Fiber: 3-4g

Serving Portion: 1 slice

Prep Time: 20 minutes **Cooking Time:** 30-35 minutes

DIET RECIPE NOTE:

1. It incorporates whole grains, healthy fats from coconut oil and nuts, and natural sweetness from maple syrup and applesauce. It avoids refined sugars, unhealthy fats, and processed ingredients that can trigger inflammation. However, be mindful of the frosting, as cream cheese and butter can be high in saturated fat. option for a lighter frosting or enjoy it in moderation.

7. Rich Carob Sheet Cake

This Rich Carob Sheet Cake offers a delicious and healthier option to local chocolate cake, making it suitable for those with RA who are looking to avoid refined sugars and potential inflammatory triggers. Carob, a naturally sweet and caffeine-free substitute for cocoa, provides a rich, chocolate-like flavor without the potential downsides. This recipe can be adapted further to enhance its RA-friendliness.

INGREDIENTS:

- 2 cups all-purpose flour

- 2 cups granulated sugar

- 2 teaspoons baking powder

- 1/2 cup carob powder

- 1/2 cup unsweetened applesauce

- 1/2 cup vegetable oil

- 1 cup water

- 1 teaspoon vanilla extract

PREPARATION METHODS:

1. Heat oven to 350°F (175°C). Grease and flour a 9x13-inch baking pan.

2. In a large bowl, mix flour, sugar, baking powder, and carob powder.

3. In a separate bowl, combine applesauce, oil, water, and vanilla extract.

4. Pour wet ingredients into dry ingredients and mix until just combined. Don't overmix.

5. Pour batter into the prepared pan and bake for 25-30 minutes, or until a toothpick inserted into the center comes out clean. 6. Let cool completely before frosting (if desired).

PREP TIPS:

1. Replace all-purpose flour with a gluten-free blend or a mix of almond and coconut flour.

2. Swap granulated sugar for coconut sugar or a natural sweetener like maple syrup (adjust liquid content if using liquid sweetener).

3. Use a heart-healthy oil like avocado or olive oil.

NUTRITIONAL VALUES PER SERVING (ASSUMING 12 SERVINGS, WITHOUT FROSTING):

Serving Portion: 1 slice

Prep Time: 15 minutes

Cooking Time: 25-30 minutes

DIET RECIPE NOTE:

The original recipe, while lower in caffeine and stimulants than a local chocolate cake, still contains refined flour and sugar, which can be inflammatory for some with RA. However, with the suggested substitutions, this cake can become a suitable treat for an RA-friendly diet. It's crucial to emphasize moderation and mindful indulgence when including any dessert, even healthier options.

_____

_____

_____

_____

_____

_____

8. Watermelon Mint Ice Pops

These refreshing and hydrating Watermelon Mint Ice Pops are a delicious treat that perfectly aligns with an RA-friendly diet. Bursting with the natural sweetness of watermelon and the invigorating touch of mint, these ice pops offer a guilt-free way to cool down and satisfy your sweet tooth. Watermelon is rich in antioxidants and vitamins, while mint adds a refreshing flavor and potential anti-inflammatory benefits.

INGREDIENTS:

- 5 cups seedless watermelon, cubed

- 1/4 cup fresh mint leaves

- 1 tablespoon lime juice (optional)

- 1-2 tablespoons honey or maple syrup (optional, adjust to taste)

PREPARATION METHODS:

1. In a blender, combine the cubed watermelon and mint leaves. Blend until smooth.

2. If desired, add lime juice and sweetener to taste. Blend again until combined.

3. Pour the mixture into popsicle molds, leaving a little space at the top for expansion.

4. Insert popsicle sticks and freeze for at least 4-6 hours or until solid.

5. To remove the popsicles from the molds, run warm water over the outside of the molds for a few seconds.

PREP TIPS:

1. If you don't have popsicle molds, you can use small paper cups and wooden sticks.

2. For a more intense mint taste, muddle the mint leaves before blending.

3. You can adjust the sweetness by adding more or less sweetener, or omit it altogether if the watermelon is sweet enough.

4. To make these popsicles vegan, use maple syrup instead of honey.

NUTRITIONAL VALUES PER SERVING (ASSUMING 6 SERVINGS):

Calories: 50-70 (depending on the sweetener used) | Protein: 1g | Carbohydrates: 12-17g | Fat: 0g | Fiber: 1g

Serving Portion: 1 ice pop

Prep Time: 10 minutes

Freezing Time: 4-6 hours

DIET RECIPE NOTE:

1. They are made with whole, unprocessed ingredients and are naturally low in fat and sodium. Watermelon is rich in lycopene, an antioxidant with potential anti-inflammatory effects.
2. Mint may also give some anti-inflammatory benefits. The optional sweetener can be adjusted or omitted based on individual liking and dietary needs.

9. Plum Cinnamon Sorbet

This Plum Cinnamon Sorbet is a delicious and refreshing dessert, perfect for individuals with rheumatoid arthritis seeking a sweet treat that aligns with their dietary needs. The natural sweetness of plums combined with the warming notes of cinnamon creates a delicious flavor profile that is both satisfying and guilt-free. This sorbet is naturally low in inflammatory triggers and offers a good source of antioxidants, making it a healthy and enjoyable dessert option.

INGREDIENTS:

- 4 cups pitted and chopped plums (about 2 pounds)

- 1/2 cup water

- 1/4 cup honey or maple syrup (adjust to taste)

- 1/2 teaspoon ground cinnamon

- 1/4 teaspoon lemon juice

PREPARATION METHODS:

1. In a medium saucepan, combine the chopped plums, water, honey (or maple syrup), and cinnamon. Bring to a simmer over medium heat, stirring occasionally.

2. Reduce heat to low and cook for 10-15 minutes, or until the plums are very soft and the mixture has thickened slightly.

3. Remove the saucepan from the heat and let cool slightly. Transfer the mixture to a blender or food processor and blend until smooth.

4. If you prefer a smoother sorbet, strain the mixture through a fine-mesh sieve to remove any remaining solids.

5. Stir in the lemon juice.

6. Pour the mixture into a freezer-safe container and freeze for at least 2 hours, or until solid.

7. Before serving, let the sorbet sit at room temperature for 5-10 minutes to soften slightly. Scoop into bowls and enjoy!

PREP TIPS:

1. For a richer taste, roast the plums in the oven at 400°F for 15-20 minutes before cooking them on the stovetop.

2. You can adjust the amount of sweetener to your liking. If the plums are very ripe and sweet, you may need less honey or maple syrup.

3. If you don't have fresh plums, you can use frozen plums. Just thaw them before using them in the recipe.

4. To make this recipe vegan, use maple syrup instead of honey.

NUTRITIONAL VALUES PER SERVING (ASSUMING 4 SERVINGS):

Calories: 150 | Carbohydrates: 35g | Fiber: 3g | Sugar: 25g (naturally occurring from fruit and added sweetener)

Serving Portion: 1/2 cup

Prep Time: 15 minutes

Cooking Time: 10-15 minutes

Freezing Time: At least 2 hours

DIET RECIPE NOTE:

1. It uses whole, unprocessed ingredients and is naturally low in fat and sodium. Plums are a good source of antioxidants, which can help fight inflammation.

2. The recipe uses natural sweeteners like honey or maple syrup, but the amount can be adjusted to taste or even omitted if the plums are very sweet.

10.   Creamy Banana Chia Pudding

Creamy Banana Chia Pudding is a delicious and nutritious breakfast or snack option, perfect for those following an RA-friendly diet. It's incredibly simple to prepare, requiring just a few wholesome ingredients, and it's rich in anti-inflammatory benefits. The chia seeds provide omega-3 fatty acids, fiber, and protein, while the banana adds natural sweetness, potassium, and antioxidants. This pudding is a delicious way to start your day or satisfy a mid-day craving.

INGREDIENTS:

- 2 ripe bananas, mashed

- 1/2 cup unsweetened almond milk (or other plant-based milk)

- 1/4 cup chia seeds

- 1 teaspoon vanilla extract

- Optional toppings: fresh berries, sliced banana, chopped nuts, cinnamon

PREPARATION METHODS:

1. In a medium bowl, combine the mashed bananas, almond milk, chia seeds, and vanilla extract.

2. Mix well until all ingredients are thoroughly combined.

3. Cover the bowl and refrigerate for at least 4 hours, or preferably overnight, to allow the chia seeds to absorb the liquid and create a pudding-like thickness.

4. Before serving, stir the pudding again to ensure it is evenly thickened.

5. Top with your desired toppings and enjoy.

PREP TIPS:

1. For a smoother texture, you can blend the bananas and almond milk before adding the chia seeds.

2. If you like a sweeter pudding, add a sprinkle of honey or maple syrup.

3. You can use any type of milk you like, but unsweetened varieties are recommended to avoid added sugars.

4. To make individual servings, divide the pudding into small jars or containers before refrigerating.

NUTRITIONAL VALUES PER SERVING (ASSUMING 4 SERVINGS):

Calories: 150 | Protein: 4g | Carbohydrates: 25g | Fat: 5g | Fiber: 7g

Serving Portion: 1/2 cup

Prep Time: 10 minutes (refrigeration time required)

DIET RECIPE NOTE:

1. This recipe is a great fit for an RA-friendly diet. It utilizes whole, unprocessed ingredients and is naturally sweetened with bananas.

2. Chia seeds provide omega-3 fatty acids, fiber, and protein, all beneficial for managing inflammation.

3. The almond milk offers a dairy-free option, suitable for those with lactose sensitivities. This recipe is also gluten-free and vegan.

11. Mixed Fruit Cobbler

A comforting and wholesome dessert, Mixed Fruit Cobbler offers a delicious way to enjoy the sweetness of fruit while adhering to an RA-friendly diet. Bursting with antioxidants and vitamins from a variety of fruits, this cobbler is a guilt-free indulgence that can satisfy your sweet tooth without triggering inflammation. The topping, made with wholesome ingredients like almond flour and coconut sugar, provides a satisfying crunch and a subtle sweetness.

INGREDIENTS:

FOR THE FILLING:

- 4 cups mixed berries (fresh or frozen)
- 1 cup chopped peaches or nectarines
- 1/4 cup coconut sugar
- 1 tablespoon lemon juice
- 1/4 teaspoon ground cinnamon

FOR THE TOPPING:

- 1 cup almond flour
- 1/2 cup rolled oats
- 1/4 cup coconut sugar
- 1/4 teaspoon baking powder
- 1/4 teaspoon salt
- 1/4 cup melted coconut oil
- 1/4 cup unsweetened applesauce

PREPARATION METHODS:

1. Heat oven to 375°F (190°C).

2. In a large bowl, combine the mixed berries, chopped peaches (or nectarines), coconut sugar, lemon juice, and cinnamon. Toss gently to coat the fruit evenly.

3. In a separate bowl, mix the almond flour, rolled oats, coconut sugar, baking powder, and salt.

4. Add the melted coconut oil and applesauce to the dry ingredients and stir until well combined. The mixture should be crumbly.

5. Transfer the fruit filling to a baking bowl (8x8 inch or similar size). Sprinkle the topping evenly over the fruit.

6. Bake for 30-35 minutes, or until the topping is golden brown and the fruit is bubbling.

7. Let cool slightly before serving. Enjoy
   warm with a dollop of coconut yogurt or
   a scoop of dairy-free ice cream (optional).

PREP TIPS:

1. Use a variety of fruits based on your liking and what's in season.

2. If using frozen fruit, there's no need to thaw it before using.

3. You can adjust the amount of coconut sugar depending on the sweetness of the fruit.

4. To make the topping gluten-free, ensure the oats are certified gluten-free.

5. Store leftovers in the refrigerator for up to 3 days.

NUTRITIONAL VALUES PER SERVING (ASSUMING 6 SERVINGS):

Calories: 300 | Protein: 5g | Carbohydrates: 40g | Fat: 18g | Fiber: 7g

Serving Portion: 1/6 of the cobbler

Prep Time: 15 minutes

Cooking Time: 30-35 minutes

DIET RECIPE NOTE:

1. This Mixed Fruit Cobbler is a suitable dessert option for individuals following an RA-friendly diet. It prioritizes whole, unprocessed ingredients like fruits, almond flour, and oats.

2. Coconut sugar offers a natural sweetener option, and coconut oil provides healthy fats. It avoids refined grains, added sugars, and unhealthy fats commonly found in local desserts. Remember that portion control is crucial when enjoying any dessert, even healthy ones!

12. Maple Almond Panna Cotta

Maple Almond Panna Cotta offers a delicious and sweet dessert that aligns beautifully with an RA-friendly diet. Its creamy texture and subtle sweetness give a satisfying end to a meal without triggering inflammation. The use of almond milk makes it a suitable option for those with lactose sensitivities, while maple syrup offers a natural sweetener with potential anti-inflammatory properties. This recipe is a testament to the fact that indulging in a delicious dessert can still be part of a healthy lifestyle.

INGREDIENTS:

- 1 3/4 cups unsweetened almond milk

- 1 packet (about 2 tsp) unflavored gelatin

- 2 tablespoons maple syrup

- 1 teaspoon pure vanilla extract

- Pinch each of ground ginger, nutmeg, and cinnamon

- 1/2 teaspoon gluten-free cornstarch (optional, for a slightly thicker texture)

- Toppings: Fresh berries, sliced almonds, a sprinkle of maple syrup

PREPARATION METHODS:

1. In a small bowl, sprinkle the gelatin over 1/4 cup of the almond milk and let it bloom for 5 minutes.

2. In a saucepan, combine the remaining almond milk, maple syrup, vanilla extract, spices, and cornstarch (if using).

3. Heat the mixture over medium heat, stirring constantly, until it comes to a simmer.

4. Remove from heat and mix in the bloomed gelatin until completely dissolved.

5. Strain the mixture through a fine-mesh sieve into a measuring cup or bowl with a spout.

6. Divide the mixture evenly among 4-6 ramekins or small glasses.

7. Refrigerate for at least 4 hours, or until set.

8. Top with fresh berries, sliced almonds, and a sprinkle of maple syrup before serving.

PREP TIPS:

1. To unmold the panna cotta, dip the ramekin in hot water for a few seconds, then run a thin knife around the edges. Carefully invert onto a serving plate.

2. If you don't have ramekins, you can use any small glasses or bowls.

3. For a vegan option, use agar agar instead of gelatin. Follow the package instructions for the correct amount.

4. Try different toppings like chopped nuts, toasted coconut flakes, or a sprinkle of cacao nibs.

NUTRITIONAL VALUES PER SERVING (ASSUMING 6 SERVINGS):

Calories: 150-180 (depending on toppings) | Protein: 3-4g | Carbohydrates: 15-20g | Fat: 10-12g

Serving Portion: 1 ramekin or small glass

Prep Time: 15 minutes

Cooking Time: 10 minutes

DIET RECIPE NOTE:

1. This Maple Almond Panna Cotta is a suitable dessert for an RA-friendly diet. It's made with whole, unprocessed ingredients and naturally sweetened with maple syrup.

2. Almond milk is a good option for those with lactose sensitivities, and the spices offer potential anti-inflammatory benefits.

3. The recipe is also gluten-free and can be easily adapted to be vegan. Remember to choose toppings that are also in line with an anti-inflammatory diet, like fresh berries and nuts.

13. Strawberry Shortcake

Strawberry shortcake is a beloved classic dessert that can be enjoyed by those following an RA-friendly diet with a few mindful adaptations. The combination of sweet, juicy strawberries and a light, fluffy cake or biscuit base offers a delicious treat without triggering inflammation. With a focus on natural sweeteners and wholesome ingredients, this dessert can be a guilt-free indulgence.

INGREDIENTS

FOR THE SHORTCAKES:

- 1 cup all-purpose flour (can be substituted with a gluten-free blend if needed)

- 1/4 cup almond flour

- 2 teaspoons baking powder

- 1/4 teaspoon baking soda

- Pinch of salt

- 1/4 cup coconut sugar or maple syrup

- 1/4 cup unsweetened applesauce

- 1/2 cup milk (dairy or plant-based)

- 1 teaspoon vanilla extract

FOR THE STRAWBERRIES:

- 2 cups fresh strawberries, hulled and sliced

- 1-2 tablespoons coconut sugar or maple syrup (adjust to taste depending on the sweetness of berries)

FOR THE TOPPING:

- 1 cup heavy cream (or coconut cream for a vegan option)

- 1 tablespoon coconut sugar or maple syrup

- 1/2 teaspoon vanilla extract

PREPARATION METHODS:

1. Heat your oven to 400°F (200°C). Line a baking sheet with parchment paper.

2. In a large bowl, mix the flour, baking powder, baking soda, salt, and coconut sugar (or maple syrup).

3. In a separate bowl, combine the applesauce, milk, and vanilla extract.

4. Pour the wet ingredients into the dry ingredients and stir until just combined. Do not overmix.

5. Drop the batter by rounded tablespoons onto the prepared baking sheet.

6. Bake for 10-12 minutes, or until golden brown and cooked through.

7. While the shortcakes are baking, combine the sliced strawberries with the coconut sugar or maple syrup in a bowl. Let sit for at least 15 minutes to macerate and release their juices.

8. In a chilled bowl, beat the heavy cream (or coconut cream) with the coconut sugar or maple syrup and vanilla extract until stiff peaks form.

9. Split each shortcake in half horizontally. Place the bottom half on a plate, and top with a generous spoonful of macerated strawberries and a dollop of whipped cream. Place the top half of the shortcake on top and enjoy!

PREP TIPS:

1. If you don't have applesauce, you can use mashed banana or an equal amount of melted coconut oil.

2. For a richer flavor, use full-fat coconut milk instead of regular milk.

3. If you prefer a crispier shortcake, bake for a few minutes longer.

4. You can also grill the shortcakes for a smoky flavor.

5. Get creative with the toppings! Add a sprinkle of chopped nuts, a drizzle of honey, or a few fresh mint leaves.

NUTRITIONAL VALUES PER SERVING (ASSUMING 4 SERVINGS):

Calories: 350-400 (depending on toppings and sweetener used) | Protein: 5-7g | Carbohydrates: 50-55g | Fat: 15-20g | Fiber: 3-4g

Serving Portion: 1 shortcake with strawberries and whipped cream

Prep Time: 20 minutes **Cooking Time:** 10-12 minutes

DIET RECIPE NOTE:

It avoids refined grains and added sugars by using whole-wheat or gluten-free flour and natural sweeteners like coconut sugar or maple syrup. The use of applesauce or mashed banana helps reduce the amount of added fat. Strawberries are rich in antioxidants, and the optional coconut cream offers a dairy-free option.

14. Baked Nut Butter Pears

This simple yet great dessert or snack is a delicious way to incorporate anti-inflammatory ingredients into your RA-friendly diet. The natural sweetness of the pears, combined with the protein and healthy fats from the nut butter, creates a satisfying and nourishing treat. Baking the pears enhances their flavor and softens their texture, making them easier to digest. This recipe is a perfect example of how healthy eating can still be delicious and enjoyable.

INGREDIENTS:

- 2 ripe but firm pears

- 2 tablespoons nut butter of choice (almond, cashew, or peanut butter)

- 1 teaspoon honey or maple syrup (optional)

- 1/4 teaspoon ground cinnamon

PREPARATION METHODS:

1. Heat oven to 350°F (175°C) and line a baking sheet with parchment paper.

2. Cut the pears in half lengthwise and scoop out the core and seeds with a spoon or melon baller.

3. In a small bowl, mix the nut butter with honey or maple syrup (if using) until smooth.

4. Fill the hollow of each pear half with the nut butter mixture.

5. Sprinkle with cinnamon.

6. Place the pears on the prepared baking sheet and bake for 20-25 minutes, or until tender when pierced with a fork.

7. Serve warm or at room temperature.

PREP TIPS:

1. Choose pears that are ripe but still firm to ensure they hold their shape during baking.

2. You can adjust the amount of nut butter and sweetener to your liking.

3. For an extra crunch, sprinkle some chopped nuts or seeds on top before baking.

4. If you don't have honey or maple syrup, you can omit it or use a sugar-free option.

NUTRITIONAL VALUES PER SERVING (2 PEAR HALVES):

Calories: 200-250 (depending on the type of nut butter and sweetener used) | Protein: 5-7g | Carbohydrates: 30-35g | Fat: 10-12g | Fiber: 5-6g

Serving Portion: 2 pear halves

Prep Time: 10 minutes

Cooking Time: 20-25 minutes

DIET RECIPE NOTE:

1. This recipe is suitable for an RA-friendly diet. It is made with whole, unprocessed ingredients and is naturally low in saturated and trans fats.
2. The pears provide fiber and antioxidants, while the nut butter offers protein and healthy fats.
3. The optional honey or maple syrup adds a touch of sweetness but can be omitted or substituted with a sugar-free option if desired.

_____

_____

_____

_____

_____

_____

_____

_____

_____

_____

_____

15. Pumpkin Pie Pot de Crème

Pumpkin Pie Pot de Crème is a delicious and comforting dessert that can be enjoyed even on an anti-inflammatory diet for managing rheumatoid arthritis. This creamy and luscious treat captures the essence of pumpkin pie without the heavy crust, making it a lighter and more digestible option. The natural sweetness of pumpkin, combined with warming spices, creates a satisfying and guilt-free indulgence.

INGREDIENTS:

- 1 cup heavy cream (or a full-fat plant-based option like coconut cream)

- 1/4 cup maple syrup (or adjust to taste)

- 1 cup pumpkin puree (not pumpkin pie mix)

- 1 teaspoon ground cinnamon

- 1/2 teaspoon ground ginger

- 1/4 teaspoon ground nutmeg

- Pinch of ground cloves

- Pinch of salt

- 3 large egg yolks

PREPARATION METHODS:

1. Heat oven to 325°F (165°C).

2. In a medium saucepan, combine heavy cream, maple syrup, pumpkin puree, cinnamon, ginger, nutmeg, cloves, and salt. Heat over medium heat, stirring constantly, until the mixture is hot and the spices are aroma, but do not boil.

3. In a separate bowl, mix the egg yolks until smooth.

4. Temper the egg yolks by slowly mixing in a small amount of the hot cream mixture. Gradually add the tempered yolks back into the saucepan with the remaining cream mixture, mixing constantly.

5. Cook over low heat, stirring constantly, until the mixture thickens and coats the back of a spoon. (It should reach about 170-175°F on an instant-read thermometer.) Do not let it boil.

6. Strain the mixture through a fine-mesh sieve into a pitcher or bowl.

7. Divide the mixture evenly among four ramekins or small bowls.

8. Place the ramekins in a baking pan and fill the pan with hot water to create a water bath (bain-marie), reaching about halfway up the sides of the ramekins.

9. Bake for 30-35 minutes, or until the custards are set around the edges but still slightly jiggly in the center.

10. Remove the ramekins from the water bath and let cool completely on a wire rack.

11. Cover and refrigerate for at least 4 hours, or preferably overnight, before serving.

12. Garnish with a dollop of whipped cream (or coconut whipped cream) and a sprinkle of cinnamon, if desired.

PREP TIPS:

1. Use high-quality spices for the best taste.

2. Make sure the egg yolks are fully incorporated into the cream mixture to avoid curdling.

3. Don't overbake the custards, or they will become dry and rubbery.

4. If you don't have ramekins, you can use small oven-safe bowls or jars.

NUTRITIONAL VALUES PER SERVING (ASSUMING 4 SERVINGS):

Calories: 300-350 (depending on the type of cream used and toppings) | Protein: 5-7g | Carbohydrates: 30-35g | Fat: 20-25g

Serving Portion: 1 ramekin

Prep Time: 20 minutes

Cooking Time: 30-35 minutes

DIET RECIPE NOTE:

It contains anti-inflammatory ingredients like pumpkin and spices, and the natural sweetness from maple syrup is preferable to refined sugar.

1. The heavy cream is high in saturated fat, which some individuals with RA may need to limit. You can substitute it with a full-fat plant-based milk alternative like coconut cream, but the texture may be slightly different.

2. While maple syrup is a better choice than refined sugar, it's still a source of sugar and should be consumed in moderation. Adjust the amount to taste or consider using a sugar substitute if needed.

3. The richness of this dessert means it's best enjoyed in smaller portions.

Self-Reflection Questions:

1. What are my current snacking and dessert habits, and how do they align with an anti-inflammatory approach?

_____

_____

_____

_____

_____

_____

2. Which RA-friendly dessert and snack recipes appeal to me the most, and why?

_____

_____

_____

_____

_____

_____

3. What challenges do I face when it comes to choosing healthy snacks and desserts, especially when cravings strike or I'm feeling stressed?

_____

_____

_____

_____

_____

_____

4. How can I make snacking and enjoying desserts a more mindful and intentional experience, rather than an impulsive or emotional one?

_____

_____

_____

_____

_____

_____

5. What are my goals for incorporating more anti-inflammatory snacks and desserts into my routine, and how will I measure my progress and celebrate my successes?

_____

_____

_____

_____

_____

_____

CHAPTER 7:
ARTHRITIS DIET SMOOTHIE RECIPES

1. "Chocolate"-Avocado Smoothie

This "Chocolate"-Avocado Smoothie is a delicious and nutritious way to start your day or refuel after a workout. The combination of creamy avocado, rich cocoa powder, and natural sweetness from fruit creates a satisfying and healthy treat. Avocado provides healthy fats, fiber, and potassium, while cocoa powder is packed with antioxidants that can help fight inflammation. This smoothie is a delicious and fulfilling option for individuals with rheumatoid arthritis.

INGREDIENTS:

- 1/2 ripe avocado, pitted and peeled

- 1 frozen banana

- 1 cup unsweetened almond milk (or other non-dairy milk)

- 2 tablespoons unsweetened cocoa powder

- 1 tablespoon maple syrup (or adjust to taste)

- 1/2 teaspoon vanilla extract

- Optional: a handful of spinach or kale for an extra boost of nutrients

PREPARATION METHODS:

1. Combine all ingredients in a blender and blend until smooth and creamy.

2. If the smoothie is too thick, add more milk until you reach your desired thickness.

3. Pour into a glass and enjoy immediately.

PREP TIPS:

1. Use a ripe avocado for the best taste and texture.

2. Freeze the banana ahead of time for a chilled and thicker smoothie.

3. If you like a sweeter smoothie, add more maple syrup or another natural sweetener like honey or dates.

4. For a more boost of protein, add a scoop of your favorite protein powder.

5. You can also add a handful of ice cubes for a colder smoothie.

NUTRITIONAL VALUES PER SERVING:

Calories: 300-350 | Protein: 5-7g | Carbohydrates: 40-45g | Fat: 20-25g | Fiber: 10-12g

Serving Portion: 1 smoothie

Prep Time: 5 minutes

DIET RECIPE NOTE:

1. This "Chocolate"-Avocado Smoothie is a great choice for an RA-friendly diet. It is rich in anti-inflammatory ingredients like avocado, cocoa powder, and banana.

2. The smoothie is also a good source of fiber, healthy fats, and essential vitamins and minerals. It is naturally low in saturated and trans fats and can be easily adjusted to be completely sugar-free by omitting the maple syrup or using a sugar substitute.

2. Minty Green Smoothie

This bright and refreshing Minty Green Smoothie is a powerhouse of anti-inflammatory ingredients, making it a nice addition to an RA-friendly breakfast or snack routine. It's rich in leafy greens, fruits, and healthy fats, offering a delicious and nutritious way to start your day or boost your energy levels. The mint adds a refreshing twist while also contributing potential anti-inflammatory benefits.

INGREDIENTS:

- 1 cup packed fresh spinach leaves

- 1/2 cup frozen mango chunks

- 1/2 cup frozen pineapple chunks

- 1/4 cup plain or Greek yogurt (or a dairy-free option like coconut yogurt)

- 1/4 cup unsweetened almond milk (or other milk of choice)

- 1 tablespoon fresh mint leaves

- 1/2 teaspoon grated ginger (optional)

- Optional sweetener: honey or maple syrup to taste (start with a small amount and adjust as needed)

PREPARATION METHODS:

1. Combine all ingredients in a blender and blend until smooth and creamy.

2. If the smoothie is too thick, add a little more almond milk or water until you reach the desired thickness.

3. Pour into a glass and enjoy immediately.

PREP TIPS:

1. For a colder smoothie, use frozen spinach or add a few ice cubes to the blender.

2. You can substitute the mango and pineapple with other frozen fruits like berries or bananas.

3. If you don't have fresh mint, you can use a small amount of mint extract, but start with a tiny amount as it can be overpowering.

4. To make this recipe vegan, use a plant-based yogurt and milk option.

5. If you prefer a sweeter smoothie, add a sprinkle of honey or maple syrup, but remember that added sugars should be consumed in moderation.

NUTRITIONAL VALUES PER SERVING:

Calories: 200-250 (depending on ingredients and added sweetener) | Protein: 5-7g | Carbohydrates: 40-45g | Fat: 5-8g | Fiber: 5-7g

Serving Portion: 1 smoothie

Prep Time: 5 minutes

DIET RECIPE NOTE:

1. This Minty Green Smoothie is a fantastic choice for an RA-friendly diet. It's rich in anti-inflammatory ingredients like spinach, mango, pineapple, and ginger.

2. The yogurt or dairy-free option provides protein and probiotics, which can support gut health and reduce inflammation. This smoothie is also naturally low in saturated and trans fats and can be easily adjusted to be low in sodium and added sugar.

_____

_____

_____

_____

_____

3. Creamy Pistachio Smoothie

A delicious and nutritious breakfast or snack option, the Creamy Pistachio Smoothie offers a rich, nutty flavor and a smooth, velvety texture that's both satisfying and refreshing. Pistachios, the star ingredient, provide a good source of protein, healthy fats, and fiber, making this smoothie a filling and energizing choice. Additionally, pistachios contain antioxidants and anti-inflammatory compounds, which may help alleviate symptoms of rheumatoid arthritis.

INGREDIENTS:

- 1 cup unsweetened almond milk (or other preferred milk option)

- 1/2 cup shelled pistachios (unsalted)

- 1/2 frozen banana

- 1/4 cup plain Greek yogurt (or plant-based yogurt option)

- 1 tablespoon honey or maple syrup (adjust to taste or omit for less sugar)

- 1/4 teaspoon ground cinnamon

- Pinch of salt

- Handful of ice cubes (optional)

PREPARATION METHODS:

1. Combine all ingredients in a blender.

2. Blend until smooth and creamy, adding more milk if needed to reach desired thickness.

3. Pour into a glass and enjoy immediately.

PREP TIPS:

1. Soak the pistachios in water for a few hours or overnight to soften them and make them easier to blend.

2. For a colder smoothie, use frozen pistachios or add a handful of ice cubes.

3. If you like a sweeter smoothie, add more honey or maple syrup, or use a ripe banana.

4. You can also add a handful of spinach or kale for an extra boost of nutrients.

5. To make this recipe vegan, use a plant-based yogurt and sweetener.

NUTRITIONAL VALUES PER SERVING:

Calories: 350-400 calories | Protein: 12-15g | Carbohydrates: 40-45g | Fat: 20-25g | Fiber: 5-7g

Serving Portion: 1 large smoothie

Prep Time: 5 minutes

Cooking Time: None

DIET RECIPE NOTE:

This Creamy Pistachio Smoothie is generally a suitable option for an RA-friendly diet. It is rich in anti-inflammatory nutrients from pistachios, bananas, and cinnamon. The healthy fats from the pistachios and yogurt contribute to satiety and help regulate blood sugar levels.

1. The natural sugars from the banana and added sweetener can contribute to the overall sugar content. Adjust the sweetener to taste or omit it altogether if you prefer.

2. If you have lactose intolerance or sensitivity, option for a plant-based yogurt option.

4. Tropical Red Smoothie

This bright and refreshing Tropical Red Smoothie is a delicious way to start your day or enjoy a healthy snack while managing rheumatoid arthritis. Bursting with antioxidant-rich berries, tropical fruits, and a hint of ginger for its anti-inflammatory properties, this smoothie provides a delicious dose of essential vitamins, minerals, and fiber. It's a quick and easy recipe that can be customized to your taste and dietary needs.

INGREDIENTS:

- 1 cup frozen mixed berries (strawberries, raspberries, blueberries)

- 1/2 cup chopped mango (fresh or frozen)

- 1/2 cup chopped pineapple (fresh or frozen)

- 1/2 cup unsweetened coconut milk (or other plant-based milk)

- 1/2-inch piece of fresh ginger, peeled and grated (optional)

- 1 tablespoon chia seeds (optional, for added fiber and omega-3s)

- Honey or maple syrup to taste (optional, if additional sweetness is desired)

PREPARATION METHOD:

1. Combine all ingredients in a blender and blend until smooth and creamy.

2. If the smoothie is too thick, add a little more coconut milk or water until you reach the desired thickness.

3. Taste and adjust sweetness with honey or maple syrup if needed.

4. Pour into a glass and enjoy immediately.

PREP TIPS:

1. Use frozen fruit for a chilled and refreshing smoothie.

2. If you don't have fresh ginger, you can omit it or use a pinch of ground ginger.

3. To make this smoothie vegan, use a plant-based milk and sweetener.

4. Add a handful of spinach or kale for an extra boost of nutrients.

5. You can also add a scoop of protein powder for a more filling smoothie.

NUTRITIONAL VALUES PER SERVING:

Calories: 250-300 (depending on added sweetener) | Protein: 5-7g | Carbohydrates: 40-45g | Fat: 10-12g | Fiber: 5-7g

Serving Portion: 1 large smoothie

Prep Time: 5 minutes

DIET RECIPE NOTE:

1. This Tropical Red Smoothie is an excellent choice for an RA-friendly diet. It's rich in antioxidants from berries and tropical fruits, which help fight inflammation.
2. The ginger adds another layer of anti-inflammatory benefits. The smoothie is naturally low in saturated and trans fats and can be easily adjusted to be sugar-free. It is also gluten-free and vegan-friendly.

_____

_____

_____

_____

_____

_____

_____

_____

_____

5. Apple-Honey Smoothie

A simple yet satisfying breakfast or snack option, this Apple-Honey Smoothie is a healthy way to incorporate anti-inflammatory ingredients into your RA diet. Apples, rich in fiber and antioxidants, provide a natural sweetness and a boost of vitamins. Honey adds a touch of additional sweetness and potential antibacterial and anti-inflammatory benefits. This smoothie is a quick and easy way to nourish your body and start your day on the right foot.

INGREDIENTS:

- 1 medium apple, cored and chopped (skin on for extra fiber)

- 1/2 cup unsweetened almond milk (or other preferred milk option)

- 1/2 frozen banana

- 1 tablespoon honey (adjust to taste or omit if desired)

- 1/4 teaspoon ground cinnamon (optional)

- Pinch of nutmeg (optional)

- Ice cubes (optional, for a thicker smoothie)

PREPARATION METHODS:

1. Combine all ingredients in a blender and blend until smooth.

2. If desired, add a few ice cubes and blend again for a chilled and thicker smoothie.

3. Pour into a glass and enjoy immediately.

PREP TIPS:

1. Use a ripe banana for natural sweetness.

2. You can adjust the amount of honey based on your sweetness likeness.

3. For an option, add a handful of spinach or kale for a more boost of nutrients.

4. If you don't have almond milk, you can use any other unsweetened milk option like oat milk or soy milk.

NUTRITIONAL VALUES PER SERVING:

Calories: 200-250 (depending on the size of the apple and the amount of honey used) | Protein: 3-5g | Carbohydrates: 40-50g | Fat: 5-7g | Fiber: 4-6g

Serving Portion: 1 smoothie

Prep Time: 5 minutes

DIET RECIPE NOTE:

This Apple-Honey Smoothie is suitable for an RA-friendly diet. It features whole, unprocessed ingredients and is naturally sweetened with fruit and honey. Apples are rich in antioxidants and fiber, while honey offers potential anti-inflammatory benefits. The smoothie is also dairy-free and gluten-free.

1. While honey has potential benefits, it's still a form of sugar and should be consumed in moderation, especially for individuals managing blood sugar levels.

2. Although natural, the fructose in fruits can contribute to overall sugar intake. It's best to enjoy this smoothie as part of a balanced breakfast or snack and not solely rely on it for your nutritional needs.

6. Vibrant Beet and Strawberry Smoothie

This bright Beet and Strawberry Smoothie is a refreshing and nutritious way to start your day or enjoy it as a healthy snack. The combination of earthy beets, sweet strawberries, and creamy bananas creates a delicious taste profile, while the addition of chia seeds boosts the nutritional value of omega-3 fatty acids and fiber. This smoothie is a powerhouse of antioxidants, vitamins, and minerals, making it an excellent addition to an anti-inflammatory diet for individuals with rheumatoid arthritis.

INGREDIENTS:

- 1 cup frozen or fresh strawberries

- 1 small beet, peeled and chopped (or 1/2 cup pre-cooked beets)

- 1 ripe banana, peeled and sliced (frozen banana adds extra creaminess)

- 1 tablespoon chia seeds

- 1 cup unsweetened almond milk (or other plant-based milk)

- Optional: a squeeze of fresh lemon juice for extra tanginess

PREPARATION METHODS:

1. Combine all ingredients in a blender and blend until smooth.

2. If the smoothie is too thick, add more almond milk or water until you reach the desired thickness.

3. Pour into a glass and enjoy immediately.

PREP TIPS:

1. For a colder smoothie, use frozen strawberries and bananas.

2. If you don't have fresh beets, you can use pre-cooked beets or roast your beets beforehand.

3. You can adjust the amount of chia seeds based on your choice.

4. Add a handful of spinach or kale for an extra boost of nutrients.

5. If you like a sweeter smoothie, add a sprinkle of honey or maple syrup, but remember to keep added sugars to a minimum.

NUTRITIONAL VALUES PER SERVING:

Calories: 250-300 (depending on ingredients and serving size) | Protein: 5-7g | Carbohydrates: 40-45g | Fat: 5-8g | Fiber: 5-7g

Serving Portion: 1 large glass

Prep Time: 5 minutes

DIET RECIPE NOTE:

1. This bright Beet and Strawberry Smoothie is a great choice for an RA-friendly diet. It is rich in anti-inflammatory ingredients, including beets, strawberries, and chia seeds. Beets are rich in betalains, potent antioxidants that have been shown to reduce inflammation.
2. Strawberries are a good source of vitamin C and other antioxidants, while chia seeds offer omega-3 fatty acids and fiber. The smoothie is naturally low in saturated and trans fats and does not contain any refined grains or added sugars (unless you choose to add a sweetener).

7. Blueberry Power Smoothie

This bright and refreshing Blueberry Power Smoothie is a perfect addition to an RA-friendly breakfast or snack routine. It's a quick and easy way to rich in antioxidants, vitamins, fiber, and protein, all essential for managing inflammation and supporting overall health. The combination of blueberries, bananas, and Greek yogurt creates a creamy and satisfying texture, while the subtle sweetness from honey (or an alternative) makes it a delightful treat to start your day or fuel your afternoon.

INGREDIENTS:

- 1 cup frozen blueberries

- 1/2 frozen banana

- 1/2 cup plain Greek yogurt (or plant-based yogurt alternative)

- 1/2 cup milk (or unsweetened plant-based milk alternative)

- 1 tablespoon almond butter (or other nut or seed butter)

- 1 teaspoon honey (or alternative sweetener to taste, such as maple syrup or stevia)

- Optional: a handful of spinach or kale for an extra boost of nutrients

PREPARATION METHODS:

1. Combine all ingredients in a blender.

2. Blend until smooth and creamy.

3. If the smoothie is too thick, add more milk or water until you reach the desired thickness.

4. Pour into a glass and enjoy immediately.

PREP TIPS:

1. For a colder smoothie, add a few ice cubes to the blender.

2. Use frozen fruit for a thicker and more refreshing smoothie.

3. If you don't have almond butter, you can use another nut or seed butter, or omit it altogether.

4. Try different sweeteners or omit them altogether if you prefer a less sweet smoothie.

5. You can add a scoop of protein powder for an extra protein boost.

NUTRITIONAL VALUES PER SERVING:

Calories: 300-350 (depending on ingredients and additions) | Protein: 15-20g | Carbohydrates: 40-45g | Fat: 10-15g | Fiber: 5-7g

Serving Portion: 1 large smoothie

Prep Time: 5 minutes

DIET RECIPE NOTE:

1. This Blueberry Power Smoothie is a great choice for an RA-friendly diet. It is rich in anti-inflammatory ingredients such as blueberries, bananas, and almond butter.
2. Greek yogurt provides a good source of protein and probiotics, which can help support gut health and reduce inflammation.
3. The smoothie is naturally low in saturated and trans fats and can be easily adapted to be dairy-free or vegan by using plant-based options for yogurt and milk. It is also a good source of vitamins, minerals, and antioxidants.

_____

_____

_____

_____

_____

_____

8. Strawberry-Mango-Banana Smoothie

A bright and refreshing start to your day, this Strawberry-Mango-Banana Smoothie is packed with vitamins, antioxidants, and fiber, making it an great choice for individuals with rheumatoid arthritis. The combination of berries, mango, and banana offers a delightful sweetness while providing essential nutrients to combat inflammation and support overall health.

INGREDIENTS:

- 1 cup frozen strawberries

- 1 cup frozen mango chunks

- 1 banana, sliced and frozen

- 1/2 cup plain or Greek yogurt (or a dairy-free option like almond or coconut yogurt)

- 1/2 cup unsweetened almond milk (or other milk of choice)

- Optional: 1 tablespoon honey or maple syrup (if additional sweetness is desired)

- Optional: 1 tablespoon chia seeds or flaxseeds (for added fiber and omega-3s)

PREPARATION METHOD:

1. Combine all ingredients in a blender and blend until smooth and creamy.

2. If the smoothie is too thick, add more almond milk or water until the desired thickness is reached.

3. Pour into a glass and enjoy immediately.

PREP TIPS:

1. Freeze the fruits in advance for a chilled and refreshing smoothie.

2. You can adjust the amount of yogurt and milk to achieve your preferred thickness.

3. If you like a sweeter smoothie, add a tablespoon of honey or maple syrup.

4. For a boost of nutrients and fiber, add a tablespoon of chia seeds or flaxseeds.

5. Feel free to try with other fruits and vegetables, such as spinach or kale, for an added nutritional punch.

NUTRITIONAL VALUES PER SERVING:

Calories: 250-300 (depending on ingredients and serving size) | Protein: 8-10g | Carbohydrates: 45-50g | Fat: 5-8g | Fiber: 5-7g

Serving Portion: 1 large smoothie

Prep Time: 5 minutes

DIET RECIPE NOTE:

1. This smoothie is a great choice for an RA-friendly diet. It's rich in anti-inflammatory fruit, providing essential vitamins, minerals, and antioxidants.
2. The yogurt offers protein and probiotics, which can support gut health and immune function. This recipe is naturally low in saturated and trans fats and can be easily adapted to be dairy-free or vegan by using plant-based options.
3. It's a delicious and nutritious way to start your day or enjoy as a refreshing snack.

_____

_____

_____

_____

_____

CHAPTER 8:
30-DAY MEAL PLAN FOR FIGHTING INFLAMMATION

Day 1:

- **Breakfast**: Omelet with Spinach and Feta

- **Lunch**: Kale and Pumpkin Seed–Stuffed Portobello Mushrooms

- **Dinner**: Spiced Trout and Vegetable Packets

- **Snack/Dessert:** Blackberry-Lemon Granita

Day 2:

- **Breakfast**: Fruit-and-Seed Breakfast Bars

- **Lunch**: Sweet Potato and Black Bean Enchiladas

- **Dinner**: Spinach Salad with Salmon and Avocado

- **Snack/Dessert:** Almond-Quinoa Crisps

Day 3:

- **Breakfast**: Chia-Coconut Porridge

- **Lunch**: Wild Rice Quinoa Salad with Grilled Vegetables and Feta

- **Dinner**: Herb and Walnut–Crusted Pork Chops

- **Snack/Dessert:** Creamy Banana Chia Pudding

Day 4:

- **Breakfast**. Mini Broccoli Frittatas

- **Lunch**: Zucchini and Avocado with Coconut-Lime Dressing

- **Dinner**: Caribbean Fish Stew

- **Snack/Dessert**: Tangy Lemon Mousse

Day 5:

- **Breakfast**: Egg Casserole with Sweet Potato and Kale

- **Lunch**: Sautéed Kale with Garlic

- **Dinner**: Spicy Shrimp Veggie Noodle Soup

- **Snack/Dessert**: Baked Nut Butter Pears

Day 6:

- **Breakfast**: Blueberry Oatmeal Bowl

- **Lunch**: Chickpea and Spinach Quesadilla–Cauliflower Pilaf

- **Dinner**: Summer Fruit, Crab, and Arugula Salad with Mint Dressing

- **Snack/Dessert**: Watermelon Mint Ice Pops

Day 7:

- **Breakfast**: Sweet Potato–Ground Turkey Hash

- **Lunch**: Grilled Eggplant and Zucchini Sandwiches

- **Dinner**: Lamb Burgers with Papaya Salsa

- **Snack/Dessert:** Plum Cinnamon Sorbet

Day 8:

- **Breakfast**: Overnight "Porridge" with Banana

- **Lunch**: Cream of Watercress and Spinach Soup

- **Dinner**: Halibut with Gingered Slaw and Avocado

- **Snack/Dessert**: Mixed Fruit Cobbler

Day 9:

- **Breakfast**: Almond Maple Muffins

- **Lunch**: Sweet Potatoes Stuffed with Lentils, Kale, and Sunflower Seeds

- **Dinner**: Shrimp Pad Thai

- **Snack/Dessert**: Strawberry Shortcake

Day 10:

- **Breakfast**: Seeds and Fruit Granola

- **Lunch**: Moroccan Parsnip Carrot Slaw

- **Dinner**: Taco Bowl with Cauliflower Rice and Avocado

- **Snack/Dessert**: Maple Almond Panna Cotta

Day 11:

- **Breakfast**: Quinoa Breakfast Bowl

- **Lunch**: Herbed Lettuce Rolls with Peach Sauce

- **Dinner**: Almond-Crusted Halibut

- **Snack/Dessert**: Pumpkin Pie Pot de Crème

Day 12:

- **Breakfast**: Lemon Vanilla Pancakes

- **Lunch**: Broiled Salmon with Lemon and Herbs

- **Dinner**: Spiced Grilled Chicken with Cauliflower "Rice" Tabbouleh

- **Snack/Dessert**: Rich Carob Sheet Cake

Day 13:

- **Breakfast**: Spinach and Mushroom Frittata

- **Lunch**: Asparagus and Beet Greens with Sesame Dressing

- **Dinner**: Italian Sausage and Kale Soup

- **Snack/Dessert**: Blueberry-Fig Open-Face Pie

Day 14:

- **Breakfast**: Salmon and Vegetable Frittata

- **Lunch**: Chicken Celeriac Chili

- **Dinner**: Shrimp and Asparagus Skillet

- **Snack/Dessert**: Berry-Rhubarb Cobbler

Day 15:

- **Breakfast**: Omelet with Spinach and Feta

- **Lunch**: Sweet Potato Sauerkraut Colcannon

- **Dinner**: Coconut and Saffron Mussel Soup

- **Snack/Dessert**: Maple Carrot Cake

Day 16:

- **Breakfast**: Quinoa Breakfast Bowl

- **Lunch**: Kale and Pumpkin Seed–Stuffed Portobello Mushrooms

- **Dinner**: Spiced Trout and Vegetable Packets

- **Snack/Dessert**: Tangy Lemon Mousse

Day 17:

- **Breakfast**: Mini Broccoli Frittatas

- **Lunch**: Sweet Potato and Black Bean Enchiladas

- **Dinner**: Herb and Walnut–Crusted Pork Chops

- **Snack/Dessert**: Creamy Banana Chia Pudding

Day 18:

- **Breakfast**: Egg Casserole with Sweet Potato and Kale

- **Lunch**: Wild Rice Quinoa Salad with Grilled Vegetables and Feta

- **Dinner**: Spinach Salad with Salmon and Avocado

- **Snack/Dessert**: Baked Nut Butter Pears

Day 19:

- **Breakfast**: Blueberry Oatmeal Bowl

- **Lunch**: Zucchini and Avocado with Coconut-Lime Dressing

- **Dinner**: Caribbean Fish Stew

- **Snack/Dessert**: Watermelon Mint Ice Pops

Day 20:

- **Breakfast**: Sweet Potato–Ground Turkey Hash

- **Lunch**: Sautéed Kale with Garlic

- **Dinner**: Spicy Shrimp Veggie Noodle Soup

- **Snack/Dessert**: Plum Cinnamon Sorbet

Day 21:

- **Breakfast**: Overnight "Porridge" with Banana

- **Lunch**: Chickpea and Spinach Quesadilla–Cauliflower Pilaf

- **Dinner**: Summer Fruit, Crab, and Arugula Salad with Mint Dressing

- **Snack/Dessert**: Mixed Fruit Cobbler

Day 22:

- **Breakfast**: Almond Maple Muffins

- **Lunch**: Grilled Eggplant and Zucchini Sandwiches

- **Dinner**: Lamb Burgers with Papaya Salsa

- **Snack/Dessert**: Strawberry Shortcake

Day 23:

- **Breakfast**: Seeds and Fruit Granola

- **Lunch**: Cream of Watercress and Spinach Soup

- **Dinner**: Halibut with Gingered Slaw and Avocado

- **Snack/Dessert**: Maple Almond Panna Cotta

Day 24:

- **Breakfast**: Quinoa Breakfast Bowl

- **Lunch**: Sweet Potatoes Stuffed with Lentils, Kale, and Sunflower Seeds

- **Dinner**: Shrimp Pad Thai

- **Snack/Dessert**: Pumpkin Pie Pot de Crème

Day 25:

- **Breakfast**: Lemon Vanilla Pancakes

- **Lunch**: Moroccan Parsnip Carrot Slaw

- **Dinner**: Taco Bowl with Cauliflower Rice and Avocado

- **Snack/Dessert**: Rich Carob Sheet Cake

Day 26:

- **Breakfast**: Spinach and Mushroom Frittata

- **Lunch**: Herbed Lettuce Rolls with Peach Sauce

- **Dinner**: Almond-Crusted Halibut

- **Snack/Dessert**: Blueberry-Fig Open-Face Pie

Day 27:

- **Breakfast**: Salmon and Vegetable Frittata

- **Lunch**: Broiled Salmon with Lemon and Herbs

- **Dinner**: Spiced Grilled Chicken with Cauliflower "Rice" Tabbouleh

- **Snack/Dessert**: Berry-Rhubarb Cobbler

Day 28:

- **Breakfast**: Omelet with Spinach and Feta

- **Lunch**: Asparagus and Beet Greens with Sesame Dressing

- **Dinner**: Italian Sausage and Kale Soup

- **Snack/Dessert**: Maple Carrot Cake

Day 29:

- **Breakfast**: Fruit-and-Seed Breakfast Bars

- **Lunch**: Chicken Celeriac Chili

- **Dinner**: Shrimp and Asparagus Skillet

- **Snack/Dessert**: Blackberry-Lemon Granita

Day 30:

- **Breakfast**: Chia-Coconut Porridge

- **Lunch**: Sweet Potato Sauerkraut Colcannon

- **Dinner**: Coconut and Saffron Mussel Soup

- **Snack/Dessert**: Almond-Quinoa Crisps

Measurement Chart

Volume Conversions

US	Metric
1 teaspoon	5 ml
1 tablespoon	15 ml
1/4 cup	60 ml
1/3 cup	80 ml
1/2 cup	120 ml
2/3 cup	160 ml
3/4 cup	180 ml
1 cup	240 ml
1 pint	473 ml
1 quart	946 ml
1 gallon	3.78 L

Weight Conversions

US	Metric
1 ounce	28 g
1/4 pound	113 g
1/2 pound	227 g
3/4 pound	340 g
1 pound	454 g

Oven Temperature Conversions

Fahrenheit (°F)	Celsius (°C)	Gas Mark
250	120	1/2
275	140	1
300	150	2
325	165	3
350	175	4
375	190	5
400	200	6
425	220	7
450	230	8
475	245	9
500	260	10

CHAPTER 9:
LIFESTYLE TIPS FOR MANAGING RHEUMATOID ARTHRITIS

The Importance of Exercise and Physical Activity

While eating healthy is a big part of managing rheumatoid arthritis (RA), it's important to remember that taking care of yourself goes beyond just food. Exercise and being active, which people with RA sometimes avoid or are scared of, are really important for keeping your joints healthy, making pain less, and improving your overall quality of life.

It's normal to feel a bit worried about exercise when your joints are inflamed and hurt. The thought of hard workouts or high-impact activities might seem too much, or even impossible. But the truth is, moving your body is like medicine for RA.

Regular exercise helps in many ways:

1. **It makes pain and stiffness less:** Exercise strengthens the muscles around your joints, giving them better support and putting less stress on the areas that hurt. It also helps your joints move more easily and through a wider range, making everyday tasks simpler.

2. **It makes you feel happier and less stressed:** Exercise releases endorphins, which are natural mood boosters that can help fight feelings of sadness and anxiety that often come with RA. It also gives you a healthy way to deal with stress and frustration.

3. **It gives you more energy:** It might sound strange, but regular exercise can make you feel less tired, which is a common problem with RA.

4. **It helps you sleep better:** Being active can help you fall asleep faster and have a more restful sleep, which is important for managing RA symptoms and staying healthy overall.

5. **It makes your bones stronger:** Exercise, especially activities that put weight on your bones, helps keep them strong and lowers the risk of osteoporosis, which is a problem that can happen with RA.

6. **It helps you keep a healthy weight:** Extra weight puts more stress on your joints, making pain and inflammation worse. Regular exercise helps you manage your weight and take some of the pressure off your joints.

The key is to find activities that you enjoy and that are right for your fitness level and how your RA is feeling at the moment. It's important to start slowly and gradually do more as you get stronger and can handle more.

Exercises that are easy on your joints, like walking, swimming, biking, and tai chi, are often recommended for people with RA. These activities give you a good workout without putting too much stress on your joints. Strength training exercises, using light weights or resistance bands, can also be helpful. These exercises help build muscle and make your joints more stable, which reduces pain and helps you move better.

Making exercise a regular part of your RA management plan can make a big difference in how you feel physically and emotionally. It's a great way to take control of your health, make pain less, move better, and improve your overall quality of life. So put on your sneakers, grab your swimsuit, or get out your yoga mat, and embrace the power of movement.

The Role of Sleep in Managing Inflammation:

Sleep is like a quiet conductor, guiding all the important things our bodies do to stay healthy. When you have rheumatoid arthritis (RA), sleep isn't just about taking a break from the day; it's a really important part of controlling inflammation and helping your body heal.

Think of sleep like a gentle wave, washing over you and taking away the stress and tiredness of the day. As you fall asleep, your body starts an amazing process of fixing and renewing itself. Your muscles relax, your tissues mend, and your immune system resets, getting ready for the next day.

If you have RA, this nighttime process is even more important. Inflammation, which is the main problem with this disease, can mess up your sleep, creating a cycle of pain, tiredness, and more inflammation. When you don't sleep well, your body can't control its immune response as well, and inflammation can get out of hand.

Studies have shown a strong link between poor sleep and worse RA symptoms. People who have trouble sleeping, like with insomnia or sleep apnea, often say they have more pain, stiffness, and tiredness. Not getting enough sleep can also make the emotional side of RA harder, leading to anxiety, depression, and feeling down.

But sleep and inflammation affect each other. Just like bad sleep can make RA worse, making sure you get good sleep can help a lot with inflammation and your overall health.

When you're in deep sleep, your body releases hormones that control the immune system and help fix tissues. Growth hormone, for example, helps muscles, bones, and other tissues grow and repair themselves. Melatonin, the sleep hormone, also fights inflammation and acts as an antioxidant.

Enough sleep also lets your body save energy and lower stress, which are both key for managing RA. When you're well-rested, you're better able to deal with the physical and emotional challenges of the disease, leading to a better mood, more resilience, and feeling more in control.

So, how can you use sleep to help manage your RA? It starts with making sleep a priority and following good sleep habits.

1. Create a calming routine before bed, without electronics or anything that gets you excited. Dim the lights, take a warm bath, or listen to relaxing music to tell your body it's time to rest.

2. Make sure your bedroom is cool, dark, and quiet, so it's easy to sleep. Get a comfortable mattress and pillows that support your joints and don't put pressure on them.

3. Go to bed and wake up at the same time every day, even on weekends. This helps your body get into a regular sleep rhythm and makes your sleep more restful.

4. Watch what you eat and drink, and how much you exercise. Avoid big meals, caffeine, and alcohol before bed, as these can mess with your sleep. Regular exercise can help you sleep better but don't exercise too close to bedtime.

If you still have trouble sleeping even after trying these things, talk to your doctor. They can figure out if there's any other medical reason, like sleep apnea, that's causing your sleep problems and suggest ways to treat it.

Exercise Tips for People with Rheumatoid Arthritis

1. **Choose Low-Impact Exercises:** Option for activities like stair climbing, walking, dancing, or using elliptical trainers. These are easier on your joints compared to high-impact exercises like running or basketball. Start with a few minutes each day and gradually increase your duration. Aim for 30-60 minutes of moderate-intensity exercise most days.

2. **Strengthen Muscles and Bones:** Do resistance exercises two to three times a week to build muscle and support your joints. This also helps burn calories. Use resistance bands, weights, or machines.

3. **Swim for Fitness:** Swimming is a great way to get exercise without stressing your joints. Start slowly in a warm pool and gradually increase your swimming time to 30 minutes per session.

4. **Try Isometric Exercises:** These involve tensing and relaxing your muscles without any visible movement. They can be a good option if strength training causes joint pain.

   i. **Chest Press:** Push your palms together firmly at chest level, hold for 5 seconds, and relax. Repeat 5 times, gradually increasing the hold time to 10-15 seconds.

   ii. **Thigh Exercise:** Sit with one leg straight and the other bent. Tighten the thigh muscles of your straight leg for 6 seconds, relax, and repeat. Switch legs and gradually increase to 15 repetitions, twice a day for each leg.

   iii. **Shoulder Extension:** Stand with your back to a wall and arms at your sides. Push your arms back towards the wall, hold for 5 seconds, and relax. Repeat 10 times.

5. **Stretch Your Fingers:** Make a fist, then open and straighten your fingers as far as you can. Repeat twice a day, gradually increasing to 20 repetitions. You can also squeeze a foam or sponge ball for added resistance.

6. **Improve Flexibility with Stretching:** Include yoga in your routine for better movement. Use moist heat or warm baths before and after stretching to ease pain and stiffness. Warm up with a 10-minute walk or similar activity. Hold stretches for 30 seconds without bouncing.

i. **Wrist Stretch:** Rest your forearm on a table and let your hand hang over the edge. Gently bend your wrist up and down with your other hand. Repeat with the other hand, increasing to 20 repetitions twice a day.

ii. **Elbow Stretch:** Extend your arms parallel to the floor with your palm facing up. Gently pull your palm towards the floor with your other hand. Hold for 30 seconds. Repeat with your palm facing down.

iii. **Calf Stretch:** Face a wall and place your palms flat on it, one foot forward and one foot back. Lean forward, keeping your heels on the floor. Hold for 30 seconds and repeat three times. Switch legs and repeat.

iv. **Hip Rotation:** Sit or lie on your back with feet slightly apart. Bend your knees inward and touch your toes together, hold for 5 seconds. Then, turn your legs and knees outward and hold for 5 seconds. Repeat twice a day, gradually increasing to 20 repetitions.

7. **Balance Rest and Exercise:** Include a mix of aerobic, strength, and flexibility exercises in your routine. Aim for at least 150 minutes of moderate-intensity aerobic exercise per week, along with two days of strength training and flexibility exercises.

8. **Avoid High-Impact Exercise:** Choose low-impact exercises like swimming, cycling, or walking to minimize joint stress. Adjust the intensity based on your fitness level and comfort.

9. **Consider Tai Chi:** This gentle martial art combines slow movements and deep breathing. Start with 10-15 minutes per session and gradually increase the duration. Aim for regular practice, ideally several times a week.

Date: _____

Monday:_____
_____
_____

Tuesday:_____
_____
_____

Wednesday:_____
_____
_____

Thursday:_____
_____
_____

Friday:_____
_____
_____

Saturday:_____
_____
_____

Sunday:_____
_____
_____

Exercise/Observation:_____
_____
_____
_____

CHAPTER 10:
14-DAY EXERCISE PLAN FOR RHEUMATOID ARTHRITIS PATIENTS

Day 1:

- 30-minute brisk walk

- 10 minutes of gentle stretching (focus on wrists, elbows, and calves)

Day 2:

- Water aerobics or swimming for 20 minutes

- Isometric exercises (chest press, thigh, shoulder extension) - 3 sets of 10 repetitions each

Day 3:

- Rest or gentle yoga for 15-20 minutes

Day 4:

- 30-minute cycling (stationary or outdoors)

- Finger stretches - 3 sets of 10 repetitions

Day 5:

- Tai Chi class for beginners (30 minutes)

Day 6:

- 45-minute walk in nature

Day 7:

- Rest or light activity like stretching or gardening

Day 8:

- Water aerobics or swimming for 30 minutes

- Isometric exercises - 3 sets of 15 repetitions each

Day 9:

- Rest or gentle yoga for 20-30 minutes

Day 10:

- 40-minute cycling

- Finger stretches - 3 sets of 15 repetitions

Day 11:

- Tai Chi class (30 minutes)

- Wrist and elbow stretch - 3 sets of 10 repetitions each

Day 12:

- 30-minute brisk walk

- Hip rotation exercise - 3 sets of 10 repetitions

Day 13:

- Rest or enjoyable activity like dancing or playing with children/pets

Day 14:

- Gentle yoga or stretching for 30 minutes

NOTE:

1. Listen to your body: If you experience pain, stop the exercise and rest.

2. Modify as needed: Adjust the duration and intensity of exercises based on your abilities and comfort level.

3. Warm up and cool down: Always include a 5–10-minute warm-up and cool-down to prevent injuries.

4. Stay hydrated: Drink plenty of water before, during, and after exercise.

5. Use heat or cold therapy: Apply heat before exercise to loosen joints and cold after to reduce inflammation.

6. Enjoy the process: Find activities you enjoy and make exercise a fun part of your routine!

Self-Reflection Questions:

1. What are my current physical activity levels, and how do they affect my RA symptoms?

2. What types of exercise do I enjoy or feel comfortable doing, even with RA?

3. What are my specific goals for incorporating exercise into my RA management plan?

4. What challenges or barriers do I anticipate facing in sticking to an exercise routine, and how can I overcome them?

5. How can I make exercise a more enjoyable and sustainable part of my life, even on days when I'm feeling fatigued or in pain?

CONCLUSIONS

Those powerful words perfectly capture the spirit of people living with rheumatoid arthritis (RA), a long-term condition that can challenge even the strongest among us. RA may bring difficulties, but it doesn't define who we are. We are empowered to overcome the pain, find strength in tough times, and build a life that is full of energy, happiness, and purpose.

"The Rheumatoid Arthritis Cookbook for Newly Diagnosed" has been your guide on this journey, giving you knowledge, inspiration, and tasty recipes to nourish your body and mind. We've explored the complexities of RA, how food can heal, and the importance of making smart choices about what you eat.

We've learned about ingredients that fight inflammation and how they can help calm the immune system and make symptoms better. From colorful fruits and vegetables to fish with omega-3s and healthy fats, we've discovered how to add these healing foods to our everyday meals, turning our kitchens into places of wellness. In this book, we've also shared stories of people who have overcome the challenges of RA, finding strength in their resilience and hope in the power of food to change things. Their experiences show us that we're not alone and that it's possible to live a full and meaningful life even with this chronic illness.

But this cookbook is more than just recipes and stories. It's a call to action, an invitation to take a whole-body approach to managing RA. It reminds us that food isn't just something we eat to survive; it's a powerful medicine that can give our bodies energy, comfort our minds, and lift our spirits. As you finish this book, we encourage you to take its lessons with you into your kitchen and life. Remember how important whole, unprocessed foods are, the value of mindful eating, and the joy of sharing meals with loved ones.

Keep exploring new tastes, try different ingredients, and find the cooking delights that bring you happiness and nourishment. Let your kitchen be a safe place where you can create not just meals but memories, connections, and a feeling of happiness.

Don't be afraid to ask for help from your healthcare team, your family, and your community. While RA is a lifelong journey, you're not alone. Surround yourself with people who understand and support you, and remember that there's strength in being together.

Most importantly, never lose hope. There will be good and bad days, times when you feel strong, and times when you have setbacks. But with each step you take and every healthy choice you make, you're building a foundation for a brighter, healthier future.

So, go forward, armed with knowledge, empowered by your choices, and fueled by the delicious possibilities that await you. Let food be your medicine, your source of comfort, and your path to a vibrant and empowered life with RA.

Dear Readers,

From the bottom of my heart, thank you for joining me on this food journey through the *"Rheumatoid Arthritis Cookbook for Newly Diagnosed."* I wrote this book with love, hoping to help those facing a new diagnosis find happiness, good food, and healing in their kitchens.

I'm so inspired by your willingness to try these recipes and see how food can be medicine. Your trust and support mean the world to me.

As a small thank you, I have a special gift for you: [Scan the QR code to access the Audio Affirmation, e.g., a Meal Planner Journal attached to the Paperback and Hardcover]. I hope this little gift makes your cooking adventures even more fun.

Remember, you're not alone on this path. I hope this cookbook becomes a friendly guide, offering tasty recipes and a feeling of belonging.

With lots of thanks,

How to Access the Affirmation Audio

SCAM THIS TO ACCESS YOUR GIFT

MEAL PLANNER AND WORKOUT CHART

Date: _____

Monday:_____

_____

_____

Tuesday:_____

_____

_____

Wednesday:_____

_____

_____

Thursday:_____

_____

_____

Friday:_____

_____

_____

Saturday:_____

_____

_____

Sunday:_____

_____

_____

Exercise/Observation:_____

_____

_____

_____

MEAL PLANNER AND WORKOUT CHART

Date: _____

Monday:_____

_____

_____

Tuesday:_____

_____

_____

Wednesday:_____

_____

_____

Thursday:_____

_____

_____

Friday:_____

_____

_____

Saturday:_____

_____

_____

Sunday:_____

_____

_____

Exercise/Observation:_____

_____

_____

_____

MEAL PLANNER AND WORKOUT CHART

Date: _____

Monday:_____

_____

_____

Tuesday:_____

_____

_____

Wednesday:_____

_____

_____

Thursday:_____

_____

_____

Friday:_____

_____

_____

Saturday:_____

_____

_____

Sunday:_____

_____

_____

Exercise/Observation:_____

_____

_____

_____

MEAL PLANNER AND WORKOUT CHART

Date: _____

Monday:_____

_____

_____

Tuesday:_____

_____

_____

Wednesday:_____

_____

_____

Thursday:_____

_____

_____

Friday:_____

_____

_____

Saturday:_____

_____

_____

Sunday:_____

_____

_____

Exercise/Observation:_____

_____

_____

_____

MEAL PLANNER AND WORKOUT CHART

Date: _____

Monday:_____

_____

_____

Tuesday:_____

_____

_____

Wednesday:_____

_____

_____

Thursday:_____

_____

_____

Friday:_____

_____

_____

Saturday:_____

_____

_____

Sunday:_____

_____

_____

Exercise/Observation:_____

_____

_____

_____

MEAL PLANNER AND WORKOUT CHART

Date: _____

Monday:_____

_____

_____

Tuesday:_____

_____

_____

Wednesday:_____

_____

_____

Thursday:_____

_____

_____

Friday:_____

_____

_____

Saturday:_____

_____

_____

Sunday:_____

_____

_____

Exercise/Observation:_____

_____

_____

_____

MEAL PLANNER AND WORKOUT CHART

Date: _____

Monday:_____

_____

_____

Tuesday:_____

_____

_____

Wednesday:_____

_____

_____

Thursday:_____

_____

_____

Friday:_____

_____

_____

Saturday:_____

_____

_____

Sunday:_____

_____

_____

Exercise/Observation:_____

_____

_____

_____

MEAL PLANNER AND WORKOUT CHART

Date: _____

Monday:_____

_____

_____

Tuesday:_____

_____

_____

Wednesday:_____

_____

_____

Thursday:_____

_____

_____

Friday:_____

_____

_____

Saturday:_____

_____

_____

Sunday:_____

_____

_____

Exercise/Observation:_____

_____

_____

_____

MEAL PLANNER AND WORKOUT CHART

Date:_____

Monday:_____

_____

_____

Tuesday:_____

_____

_____

Wednesday:_____

_____

_____

Thursday:_____

_____

_____

Friday:_____

_____

_____

Saturday:_____

_____

_____

Sunday:_____

_____

_____

Exercise/Observation:_____

_____

_____

_____

MEAL PLANNER AND WORKOUT CHART

Date: _____

Monday:_____

_____

_____

Tuesday:_____

_____

_____

Wednesday:_____

_____

_____

Thursday:_____

_____

_____

Friday:_____

_____

_____

Saturday:_____

_____

_____

Sunday:_____

_____

_____

Exercise/Observation:_____

_____

_____

_____

MEAL PLANNER AND WORKOUT CHART

Date: _____

Monday:_____

_____

_____

Tuesday:_____

_____

_____

Wednesday:_____

_____

_____

Thursday:_____

_____

_____

Friday:_____

_____

_____

Saturday:_____

_____

_____

Sunday:_____

_____

_____

Exercise/Observation:_____

_____

_____

_____

MEAL PLANNER AND WORKOUT CHART

Date: _____

Monday: _____

_____

_____

Tuesday: _____

_____

_____

Wednesday: _____

_____

_____

Thursday: _____

_____

_____

Friday: _____

_____

_____

Saturday: _____

_____

_____

Sunday: _____

_____

_____

Exercise/Observation: _____

_____

_____

_____

MEAL PLANNER AND WORKOUT CHART

Date: _____

Monday:_____

_____

_____

Tuesday:_____

_____

_____

Wednesday:_____

_____

_____

Thursday:_____

_____

_____

Friday:_____

_____

_____

Saturday:_____

_____

_____

Sunday:_____

_____

_____

Exercise/Observation:_____

_____

_____

_____

MEAL PLANNER AND WORKOUT CHART

Date: _____

Monday:_____
_____
_____

Tuesday:_____
_____
_____

Wednesday:_____
_____
_____

Thursday:_____
_____
_____

Friday:_____
_____
_____

Saturday:_____
_____
_____

Sunday:_____
_____
_____

Exercise/Observation:_____
_____
_____
_____

MEAL PLANNER AND WORKOUT CHART

Date: _____

Monday:_____

_____

_____

Tuesday:_____

_____

_____

Wednesday:_____

_____

_____

Thursday:_____

_____

_____

Friday:_____

_____

_____

Saturday:_____

_____

_____

Sunday:_____

_____

_____

Exercise/Observation:_____

_____

_____

_____

MEAL PLANNER AND WORKOUT CHART

Date: _____

Monday:_____

_____

_____

Tuesday:_____

_____

_____

Wednesday:_____

_____

_____

Thursday:_____

_____

_____

Friday:_____

_____

_____

Saturday:_____

_____

_____

Sunday:_____

_____

_____

Exercise/Observation:_____

_____

_____

_____

MEAL PLANNER AND WORKOUT CHART

Date: _____

Monday:_____

_____

_____

Tuesday:_____

_____

_____

Wednesday:_____

_____

_____

Thursday:_____

_____

_____

Friday:_____

_____

_____

Saturday:_____

_____

_____

Sunday:_____

_____

_____

Exercise/Observation:_____

_____

_____

_____

MEAL PLANNER AND WORKOUT CHART

Date: _____

Monday:_____
_____
_____

Tuesday:_____
_____
_____

Wednesday:_____
_____
_____

Thursday:_____
_____
_____

Friday:_____
_____
_____

Saturday:_____
_____
_____

Sunday:_____
_____
_____

Exercise/Observation._____
_____
_____
_____

MEAL PLANNER AND WORKOUT CHART

Date: _____

Monday:_____

_____

_____

Tuesday:_____

_____

_____

Wednesday:_____

_____

_____

Thursday:_____

_____

_____

Friday:_____

_____

_____

Saturday:_____

_____

_____

Sunday:_____

_____

_____

Exercise/Observation:_____

_____

_____

_____

MEAL PLANNER AND WORKOUT CHART

Date: _____

Monday:_____

_____

_____

Tuesday:_____

_____

_____

Wednesday:_____

_____

_____

Thursday:_____

_____

_____

Friday:_____

_____

_____

Saturday:_____

_____

_____

Sunday:_____

_____

_____

Exercise/Observation:_____

_____

_____

_____

MEAL PLANNER AND WORKOUT CHART

Date: _____

Monday:_____

_____

_____

Tuesday:_____

_____

_____

Wednesday:_____

_____

_____

Thursday:_____

_____

_____

Friday:_____

_____

_____

Saturday:_____

_____

_____

Sunday:_____

_____

_____

Exercise/Observation:_____

_____

_____

_____

Made in the USA
Columbia, SC
28 September 2024

d4346763-c9bf-49c1-b072-90e627d75146R02